TM

Theinspirationalseries™
Overcoming adversity and thriving

The Mad Traveller

Waking up from Fugue

BY IMOGEN GROOME

We are proud to introduce The**inspirational**series™. Part of the Trigger family of innovative mental health books, The**inspirational**series™ tells the stories of the people who have battled and beaten mental health issues. For more information visit: www.triggerpublishing.com

THE AUTHOR

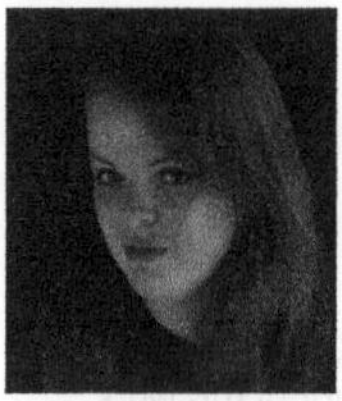

Imogen Groome is a journalist, copywriter and digital marketer living in London, England. She has worked in the creative industry for over six years, using her platform to speak out about mental health in Metro.co.uk, Huffington Post UK and more.

The Mad Traveller is Imogen's first non-fiction book. It depicts her journey through dissociative fugue, or reversible amnesia, where she experienced memory loss and lost her sense of self as a response to extreme stress and anxiety. Some of her memories are still lost, but enough have returned to form a narrative describing what it's like to lose all sense of who you are.

She has written her book in the hope that it will encourage people to speak openly about what's going on in their heads, and instill in them a belief that they can build a successful life while dealing with mental health issues.

First published in Great Britain 2019 by Trigger

Trigger is a trading style of Shaw Callaghan Ltd & Shaw Callaghan 23 USA, INC.

The Foundation Centre

Navigation House, 48 Millgate, Newark

Nottinghamshire NG24 4TS UK

www.triggerpublishing.com

British Library Cataloguing in Publication Data

A CIP catalogue record for this book is available upon request from the British Library

ISBN: 978-1-912478-70-5

This book is also available in the following e-Book and Audio formats:

MOBI: 978-1-912478-73-6

EPUB: 978-1-912478-71-2

PDF: 978-1-912478-72-9

AUDIO: 978-1-912478-74-3

Cover design and typeset by Fusion Graphic Design Ltd

Printed and bound in Great Britain by Clays Ltd, Elcograf S.p.A

Paper from responsible sources

TRIGGER™

The voice of mental health

www.triggerpublishing.com

Thank you for purchasing this book.
You are making an incredible difference.

Proceeds from all Trigger books go directly to
The Shaw Mind Foundation, a global charity that focuses
entirely on mental health. To find out more about
The Shaw Mind Foundation visit,
www.shawmindfoundation.org

MISSION STATEMENT

Our goal is to make help and support available for every single person in society, from all walks of life.
We will never stop offering hope. These are our promises.

Trigger and The Shaw Mind Foundation

the Shaw mind
FOUNDATION

Creating hope for children,
adults and families

A NOTE FROM THE SERIES EDITOR

The Inspirational range from Trigger brings you genuine stories about our authors' experiences with mental health problems.

Some of the stories in our Inspirational range will move you to tears. Some will make you laugh. Some will make you feel angry, or surprised, or uplifted. Hopefully they will all change the way you see mental health problems.

These are stories we can all relate to and engage with. Stories of people experiencing mental health difficulties and finding their own ways to overcome them with dignity, humour, perseverance and spirit.

Imogen's story is a story of our times. You don't need to have experienced dissociative fugue to relate to Imogen and the challenges she has faced. Through a life of knock-backs, bullying and hardship, it's a story that is all too familiar to many people. But what makes her story sing is her absolute commitment to keep going, against all the odds. For the first few years of her life, Imogen was running away, but as her story develops, we see Imogen taking control and winning the fight of her life.

This is our Inspirational range. These are our stories. We hope you enjoy them. And most of all, we hope that they will educate and inspire you. That's what this range is all about.

Lauren Callaghan,

Co-founder and Lead Consultant Psychologist at Trigger

To Deb, for believing in my light,
To Cam, for keeping it bright,
To Leslie, for helping me find it.

Disclaimer: Some names and identifying details have been changed to protect the privacy of individuals.

Trigger Warning: The book contains references to sexual abuse and suicide.

Trigger encourages diversity and different viewpoints, and is dedicated to telling genuine stories of people's experiences of mental health issues. However, all views, thoughts, and opinions expressed in this book are the author's own, and are not necessarily representative of Trigger as an organisation.

MISSING

The English detective novelist Agatha Christie disappeared on the evening of 3rd December 1926.

Her mother had passed away a few months previously, and her husband was having an affair which he was making little effort to keep hidden.

Agatha wrote several notes to her husband and a few others, each one telling a different story. One of them said that she was going on holiday to Yorkshire; in another, she wrote that she feared for her life.

The next morning, Agatha's car was discovered in Surrey, near a lake called Silent Pool, in which she had drowned one of her fictional characters. The headlights had been left on; the bonnet was left up. Her fur coat, an expired driving licence and a suitcase full of her belongings had been left inside the vehicle.

15,000 volunteers were gathered to search the countryside, and the police dredged the lake. In a first for England, planes were flown overhead in an effort to find the missing person. But all of their attempts were in vain. Agatha was nowhere to be found. Her disappearance made national headlines.

At a health spa in Harrogate, Yorkshire, a bereaved mother from Cape Town called Teresa Neele checked in. A few people thought they recognised her from somewhere, but eventually concluded they were clearly mistaken.

On 14th December, the police took Agatha's husband to the spa, suspecting Teresa Neele wasn't who she said she was. As he entered, Agatha remarked: 'Fancy, my brother has arrived.'

Agatha never discussed this episode. Some believe it was an act of revenge, or a publicity stunt. But her doctors had an altogether different idea. They believed it was an episode of fugue state, or dissociative fugue.

PROLOGUE

I sat in my father's front room, simultaneously feeling bored, lost, and at my wit's end. Before I knew what I was doing, I'd booked a night in a hotel and walked out of the house. I was 20 years old.

I got a train to Brighton and spent the afternoon lying on the beach, looking out at the waves. I closed my eyes and emptied my mind, then let it fill up with what surrounded me. The briny scent of the sea. The sound of the waves lapping at the shore. The hum of voices as people walked along the seafront.

When I opened my eyes, I focused on the multiple shades of grey in the rocks around me, the number of times a wave hit the shore in a five-minute interval, the sun slowly setting in the background.

I'd needed to empty my mind of everything that was cluttering it. Many of us do it – we decide we need some time away, and go somewhere quieter, to recharge.

The evening turned to night, and I decided to take a trip to the cinema. It was there that I saw the movie adaptation of John Green's *Paper Towns*, which tells the story of a shy teenager called Quentin, who is in love with the mysterious and popular Margo.

After a night of adventures together, Quentin discovers that his love has disappeared, but he knows she is off doing her own thing. Rumours about where she could be spread all over their school, but none of them are true. In reality, she is in a "paper town" in New York – a fictional town created by map makers.

When he discovered a trail of clues Margo left behind, Quentin took it upon himself to find her. But upon discovering her whereabouts, and suggesting it was time for her to return home to "normal" life, Margo said she didn't know who she was. She rejected the traditional plan of going to college, getting a job, getting married, and settling down. With two realities open to him, Quentin finally turned down the chance to join her, and returned home to his conventional life.

The film struck a chord. I had always felt stuck in a suffocating limbo between these two realities. Was I meant to get a job, find a partner, have children, and do all that traditional life stuff everyone seems to just get on with, no questions asked? Or was I meant to go wandering, exploring the world, and doing all the amazing things I dreamt of?

There were certainly times when I'd dreamt of being able to wander off somewhere and forget the life I was living. In fact, I had already done that, on many occasions, each one more painful than the last, and with more severe repercussions.

Although I could have drifted through Brighton forever – or, in theory, gone anywhere in the world and set up a life there – I got back on the train two days later and returned home. I had a father and brothers who would worry if I disappeared, and one of the things that kept me grounded, besides mindfulness techniques, was the visualisation I had in my mind of their pain, if I had gone missing again.

The urge never quite goes away though. Even now, if I'm working late, feeling tired, and idly scrolling through Facebook photos of people from high school exploring Australia on working holiday visas, I feel the drive to do the same. It's only the thought that if I do it, I won't ever come back that stops me. And deep down, I want to feel anchored somewhere. I want to belong. I want to try to walk the conventional path we're taught we have to follow.

My trip to Brighton was backed up by a fixed time frame, a text to my dad to let him know what I was doing, and a planned return home date. But my teenage years had been dominated by gaps of time that I completely lost; times when life got too difficult for my mind to deal with and I'd just switched off and walked out. Where to, I didn't know until some time afterwards. It wasn't like disappearing to a fictional town to make a new life, Margo-style. When I shut down, I forgot about my life. Sometimes I made up new identities. I was lost.

Some of my memories of those times have returned intact. Others are hazy. And a few are so harrowing I'm not sure if they're real or not.

The most disturbing part isn't having no memory of the times I wasn't myself, it's the times I experienced stuff knowing it was real ...

Being yelled at by a policewoman who was convinced I'd broken into a building, when really, I'd been hiding in it for several hours. Standing on the top of a bridge, knowing I'd been incredibly close to jumping. Drop rolling out of a stranger's car after walking 10 miles down a dual carriageway, then sleeping by the side of a road until dawn.

Knowing that I went through all of that stuff, remembering every part of my conscious experience in such vivid detail, in the immediate aftermath of each episode, is what I found hardest to shake.

Still, I will sometimes have dreams that offer snatches of evocative memories from over a decade ago. They don't just come with sights; I experience the sounds and scents from my past, too ...

The feel of a lamp outside a house in a village, hot against my freezing palm as I pressed up against it on a cold winter night. The sound of the alarms in my school, that started going off when I emerged from my hiding place, and reverberated in my ears, causing me to hide under a desk until a sniffer dog found me. The lights from the cars that drove past me as I shivered outside a barn on a pitch-black country road ... these are the impressions and scent memories that haunted me for years afterwards, and still slide into my mind every so often.

By the time I reached my early twenties, the memories my mind had blocked due to their traumatic nature had started seeping back, and the flashbacks haunted both my nights and days. They are the stories that fascinated psychiatrists, shocked friends to silence and left me feeling ... numb.

CHAPTER 1

STARTING OUT BLIND

I am lucky to be alive. I am lucky to be safe, and to be sane (although some of my friends will jokingly argue otherwise). Most of all, I am lucky to have a life that I know is my own.

To be able to look in the mirror and know who I am, what my name is, what I'm thinking and feeling, what my hopes and dreams are, what I want from life ... these are luxuries I never take for granted.

It sounds silly, right? How can I not know who I am? We come into this world with a name assigned to us, and the capacity to learn, grow, and form our own opinions. The fortunate among us live in a house in a respectable community with parents who love us, siblings who annoy us, a school down the road or a short car ride away, and we go through life like everyone else does. We know what we are meant to do, we get an education, we find a career, we settle down and have kids of our own.

But our way into the world is not always straightforward ...

The second of three children, I was born into this world blind. My mother told me she had to come to terms with the fact that first she had a son with autism and then, a blind daughter. The nurse didn't even break the news gently; she was just as stunned as my mother must have been. 'She's blind, Miriam,' she blurted out.

'I felt that I'd failed, somehow,' Mum told me one summer afternoon when I was in my late teens. 'All I wanted was this family, to have children and care for them, but suddenly I was being presented with obstacles I didn't know how to deal with.

'I was exhausted. We registered you for the blind school in Worcester. I accepted that this household would be far from normal – although what does "normal" mean, anyway? I knew that I had to really step up as a mother, to make life as good as possible for both of you.'

We don't typically remember what happened to us in our earliest years, but I remember sounds and smells. I remember being lifted up, feeling weightless, and I remember the rush of cool air on my cheeks. I remember a sweet, warm smell, which I would later associate with my mother baking in the kitchen on a Sunday afternoon. I remember the feeling of softness beneath me when it was quiet, and I turned to my dreams.

My retinas were detached, but incredibly, they attached themselves a few months later, and I was given the gift of sight. One of my first memories is of our garden. My dad was a keen gardener, and we were surrounded by flowers. There was a bench my mum would sit on, cradling me, and seeing the vivid colours surrounding me gave me a sense of calm.

As I adjusted to having sight, my mother would check on me at night and be alarmed to find me lying in bed, eyes wide open. She would call my name, and I'd wake up; I was sleeping with my eyes open, because I was not yet accustomed to having my eyes open during the day and then closing them when it was time to sleep.

I was a quiet child. So quiet, in fact, that my parents would sometimes worry there was something wrong. They had two extremes – an elder son, Tom, who was nonverbal and prone to having extreme temper tantrums, and a daughter who was content to simply sleep or sit in the corner, gazing out at the world.

In my earliest years, I would go out into the garden after my father had mowed the lawn and breathe it in, feeling a sense of utter peace. It was solace from the jumbled thoughts whirling around my head, which I could not make sense of. I would sometimes look out at the night sky, when I was lying in bed, unable to sleep, and think about what would happen if the Earth was destroyed. It could be a meteorite, or aliens, or maybe some invisible disease that silently killed us all. I would have nightmares, and visions during the day, of menacing alien faces, people burning, or rows of corpses.

To distract me from these disturbing thoughts, I would become very focused on what was around me. I would sit on the bench, feeling the slight dampness of the wood beneath me, the sound of bees buzzing their way around the flowers, and the sweet scent of the honeysuckle my father had planted. They were bright, colourful and simple, and they made me feel warm inside. They were comforting in a world I struggled to make sense of.

I would clean my teeth in the bathroom at night and gaze at my reflection in the big bathroom mirror. A tall girl with blonde hair and baby-blue eyes gazed back. I knew that reflection inside out – the smattering of freckles on the bridge of her nose, the larger ones across her cheeks, the broad shoulders and the unruly bits of fringe that curled up whenever they felt like it. But I didn't know who I was. Night after night, I stared at myself.

Why was I here? Why should I be here? What purpose did I have on this planet? Little did I know, I was asking the big questions. At the age of eight, when I should probably have been focusing on my mental arithmetic, I was having an existential crisis. All those big questions continued swirling around my brain for years. Staring into those big blue eyes that seemed to go on forever, I felt cut off from the people around me, and I didn't understand what my place in the world was. What made me, me?

I did not know. All I knew was that I had been named Imogen and I liked to read, but I was not content with just that. I wanted more. I dreamt of more. I did not think that was enough.

I quickly became an accomplished speller, and my advanced reading age meant I went to English lessons with children five years my senior. I would spend hours in my room every night, escaping to other worlds that people had created. They were easier to stomach than the confusing and disorienting world I had to face.

Some of the first books I read in school were *The Magic Key* series. I was obsessed. Biff and Chip would see the key on Floppy the dog's collar start to glow, and know they were being whisked away on a marvellous adventure. They did incredible things, saw fantastic creatures in faraway lands, then crash back into normal life with a thump and go about their everyday lives.

Whenever a new *Magic Key* book was available in school, I would eagerly stuff it into my school bag and curl up on my bed, devouring the words.

I would look out of the window at night, hoping for a magic key to float in through the window and take me away to a faraway land. I wanted to become an adventurer, to do amazing things. Maybe then, I would know who I was.

But every time I looked, the only things I saw were the row of houses in our boring cul-de-sac, the occasional glow of light from one of the rooms opposite, and sometimes one of our neighbour's dogs would come out and start yapping away in the front porch.

It was the same every time, and I felt trapped. Bored. Empty. I wanted more. I wanted to escape. To forget who I was, leave behind my dull life, and become someone exciting who did amazing things.

It was just a shame my social skills were non-existent ... Mum got me enrolled in summer schools and extracurricular activities to help me try to make friends, but I never knew what to say to other people. I had no idea how to chatter away like the other girls did. Instead, I'd make friends with one girl at a time, and preferred to sit on my own on the days she wasn't around. Teachers or assistants would try to sit me down with other kids, but I wouldn't want to talk to them, because trying to hold a conversation with more than one person felt like too much. Besides, it was much more comforting to be in my own head, because I could sit and create stories that felt much more fun than the boring activities I was supposed to do.

When I was six, my younger brother, Harry, was born, and by the time he was eight, his own autism was presenting itself. My parents were quite overprotective as a result, and Dad wouldn't let me go on residential trips with my classmates. Although I know he was trying to keep me safe, I feel that living in such a bubble as a child ultimately led to me struggling to navigate the real world when I finally entered it.

There was nothing more isolating than having to sit with the year below for a week while my classmates went on adventure holidays, or on a trip to France, then having to sit and listen to them all gushing about what they'd been up to, knowing I was outside of the picture. An outsider. Alone.

Whenever I went anywhere with the family, I felt I never got to do anything I wanted to do. I'd be going on walks with Dad, where he would browse garden shops, and I'd stand around feeling bored. Or I'd go out to Cheltenham or Stratford-upon-Avon with Mum, and she'd browse lotions in Boots, while I wandered the aisles, wanting to do anything but whatever pleased my parents or my brothers. Why couldn't I try to find out what made me happy? I felt so restrained.

By the time I was 10, the works of Jacqueline Wilson were fascinating to me, and whenever I visited a bookstore with my parents, I would beg them to buy me the latest novel. But Mum wanted me to read a broader range of books, and didn't want me obsessing over just one author. I couldn't help it, though, I was fascinated by the worlds Wilson presented in her novels.

Tracy Beaker had been left in *The Dumping Ground*, and dreamt of meeting her mum, while I sometimes wished I could have a break from mine. *The Illustrated Mum* was covered in tattoos; beautiful illustrations adorning the body that my gran would sneer at and call "common". These realities were so alien from my own, I couldn't help but greedily seek out more material to drown myself in.

It reached a point where Mum banned me from having any more, but Dad would always forget which author he couldn't buy me. 'Oh, it's J.K. Rowling who's not allowed, I have a real thing for *Harry Potter*,' I'd say, merrily trotting up to pay for another Jacqueline Wilson novel and hiding it from my mother until one day she'd discover it while cleaning and give me a thorough bollocking.

I felt like an empty shell. Like I was going through the motions, but not really living. I found classwork easy; I was top of my class, but that didn't do me any favours when it came to making friends with my peers. Largely, I was ignored. Or bullied. Being different was a threat. I knew I was different, but I didn't know what that meant.

Deep down, I had a feeling of not belonging, and wanted to find somewhere that I fitted in. Unfortunately, the road towards finding myself was one full of danger, pockets of lost time, and feeling even more lost than I ever did as a little girl.

CHAPTER 2

SUGAR PUFF MONSTER

'Oh my God, it's hit her right on the bum, look!'

Although it clearly hadn't been me they were talking to, I turned around to look and saw the girls who loved to bully me were right. The wet toilet roll had indeed hit me right on my backside. It lay, dripping, on the floor, after achieving its desired effect and slipping, wetly, to the ground.

The back of my skirt was wet, making it look like I'd had an accident – but worse, it was covered in flakes of wet toilet paper that would be a nightmare to remove.

If I wanted to get them all off before they dried, I'd be late to my next class. The group of cackling girls knew that, and, confident they'd completed their mission for the morning, they swanned back to the girls' toilets to re-apply their lip gloss.

If I went in there to clean my skirt, I'd be subjected to more cackling, sneering, and pointing. So, I decided to bypass that, and took the stairs to the toilets just outside my English class, where I could brush off the flakes as quickly as possible, then take my seat and wrap my long cardigan around my skirt for the rest of the day.

Once inside the toilets, I stepped inside a vacant cubicle and locked the door. Only then did I let a few tears roll down my cheeks. I hated school. That was a common complaint for many of my 13-year-old peers, but I didn't hate it because of the lessons or the teachers. I liked learning, and I got on better with the teachers than my fellow pupils.

No, I hated school because I was treated like an alien. I was constantly aware of how I didn't fit in. My tall, stocky figure did not match the short, slender frames of the other girls. I couldn't use hair straighteners. Mum had said I would burn myself, so my hair was constantly a frizzy mess. I wore round, Harry Potter-style glasses, and had large eyes and lips. Most of the time I chose trousers instead of skirts – being too self-conscious about my large thighs, and not wanting them to chafe when I got hot.

My shoes weren't fashionable, or from any of the high-street stores my peers went to; Mum got my shoes from whichever factory shop she'd visited lately, because they were discounted and because "You're going to grow so quickly, I may as well get you one good, sturdy pair of shoes you can rely on for years, never mind the latest fashion trends."

I was going to school to learn, not walk down a catwalk or runway. But as I sat in class each day in my bulky blazer, male button-down shirt and plain shoes, I wished I could at least pretend I was runway-ready.

I was so envious of the other girls in my year, who seemed to have a ready-made group of friends. They all wore the same accessories with their uniforms: identical flat black shoes and stylish see-through tights. Although make-up was banned, they managed to wear the right blend of mascara and lip gloss to make their facial features stand out, without being so obvious that teachers could easily pull them up on it.

One afternoon, our maths teacher had told a popular girl off for "blatantly wearing mascara", and she'd batted her eyelids in faux outrage, exclaiming, 'Sir, of course I'm not! Are you discriminating against me for having longer eyelashes?' Then he'd spluttered incoherently and looked flustered, while she waved at one of the boys, who was openly perving on her from across the room.

I was bored of school. Bored of going through the motions of lessons when I knew I'd learn it all quicker if I just read the textbooks at home. Bored of looking at all the other pupils interact with each other, and then getting bullied myself because I wasn't like them. But at the same time, I wanted so badly to be one of them, because then, maybe, it wouldn't hurt so much.

I dealt with the emptiness I felt by eating. It didn't really matter what I ate. Whenever Mum left the house to pick up one of my brothers, a strange frenzy would begin, and I would rush around the house, grabbing whatever I could find to eat that wouldn't be missed. Sometimes if there wasn't much available, I'd raid the freezer, taking out frozen flapjack and shoving it in my mouth before it defrosted, hiding the wrappers in my school bag.

It made me gain weight, and I didn't feel better in the long run, but for those few minutes I let the frenzy happen, I felt like I had control over something.

I wasn't the only one who got bullied, of course. There was a guy called Sam who was much shorter than everyone else. This gave people an obvious "in" to make him feel bad about his physical appearance, and I soon realised I was almost lucky; the worst I had to deal with on a physical level was having toilet rolls thrown at my backside.

It soon became a weekly pattern. Every week, I'd have top-set French class with Sam and a handful of the popular girls. Everyone would pile into the classroom, but there'd be one face missing.

'Where's Sam?' our teacher would ask, with a resigned look on her face. She already knew the answer.

'He's in the locker, Miss,' a few of us would chorus, and she'd let out a sigh before leaving the classroom to fetch the master key from the staff room.

Much as I imagined it was probably pretty uncomfortable, and demeaning, to be shoved into a locker every Wednesday breaktime, Sam did at least have his own group of friends at school, and they looked out for him where they could. Mostly, I was alone. And an easy target ...

There was an outdoors corridor where all the cool kids hung out, and it couldn't be avoided if you needed to walk down the stairs and get to one of the outside buildings for a class. I came to dread that corridor, because it would become a spotlight for people to have insults hurled at them.

I'd appear at the top of the stairs, and whoever was on lookout would tell the others I was coming. Then I'd brace myself and start the walk.

'Hagrid!'

This one I was used to. I was tall and fat. They thought it was witty and creative.

'Fish lips!'

I'd had this one since primary school. It was nothing new.

'Four eyes!'

The insult was so unoriginal and tired, I almost yawned when I heard it.

'Sugar Puff Monster!'

The first time I heard this, I turned around. 'What the hell does that even mean?' I asked. I couldn't help myself. I at least wanted to understand the logic behind the insults before they were hurled at me.

In a perverse way, it made me feel better if someone could justify what they were saying to me. At least I could understand the reasoning, compare it to my appearance, and go, 'Fair enough. You're a twat for saying it, but fair enough.'

The kid was thrown. 'You know, the thing on the cereal box. The monster with the blonde hair and googly eyes. You look like him, innit.'

This justification made it even more clear to his friends scattered around him, who started guffawing and pointing at me. Clearly this comparison made perfect sense, and it was hilarious. Now I knew what insult they'd be leading with from now on.

It hurt. It just ... hurt. There was no other way of describing it. I never showed them the hurt, of course. Why show them they've won? I just rolled my eyes and walked away. But inside I felt all churned up, slightly sick and, more than anything, depressed as hell. Why did this have to be my existence? I hadn't asked to be born. I hadn't asked to be here. Why was I being forced to go through life, dealing with a load of idiots each day, doing boring lessons I could complete with my eyes closed, then going home and feeling alone, with books my only solace?

While everyone else spent their mid-morning and lunch breaks in the playground, the empty classrooms, or hanging out in the fields, I would increasingly retreat to my favourite toilet cubicle and stay there until the bell rang. It was the largest cubicle, with a wall on one side and a window at the top. This helped me feel anchored, because being at school left me feeling like I'd been cast adrift, with nowhere to go.

Sometimes I'd hug the wall during my lunch break, fighting back the tears, because life felt impossible. What was the point? I knew I'd grow older and escape the monotony of school life, go to university, find a job I enjoyed, maybe settle down and find someone. But all any of it led to, in the end, was death. Why go through the façade of living a life you hadn't asked for, just to die at the end of it? Why try to be important, do something with your life, when we were all just tiny specks on a tiny ball-shaped planet in a massive universe? Our lives were just a brief, fleeting moment, compared to the history of the planet and the universe, so what did any of it mean? Why was I here? What was the fucking POINT?!

The thoughts swirled around my brain endlessly, with no answer ever rising to the surface. I thought about telling someone about what was going on in my head, but if I barely understood the thoughts myself, how the hell would anyone else make sense of them?

I felt a perpetual sense of fear due to this lack of answers about my identity. I'd been given so many labels at school. Freak. Weirdo. Loner. Hagrid. Four eyes. Sugar Puff Monster. But none of them meant anything.

I wondered if I'd have felt differently, if I'd had a group of friends. Something told me that would have made it easier, but the questions would still have remained ...

What anchored me to the identity I'd been given?

What made it so absolute for everyone else in the world?

Why did we all go through life, not questioning our names, our faces, our place in society?

What was expected of us and the dreams we were supposed to have?

I knew how to dream, but I didn't know how to be me. The concept of "me" was as fluid as the fictional realities I floated through when life was so hard to stay anchored to.

After a few years, I was pretty sick of the monotony. Waking up, listening to my brothers fight, walking through the school entrance, sitting in the toilets alone, or in classrooms feeling alone, was just bullshit. Everything was bullshit. So, I started walking out of lessons that bored me.

It confused the teachers, especially my English teacher. None of it made sense on paper. I was a quiet, conscientious pupil, who got good grades. Why was I walking out of class like the kids who didn't want to learn, when I so clearly engaged with my lessons and did well?

The answer was I felt like nobody gave a damn. So why should I keep up the routine when it was just making me feel like I was dying inside? I could almost feel myself shrivelling up like a flower past its prime, turning black, the petals dropping onto the ground, one by one.

One afternoon, an English lesson saw the class working in groups on an activity related to the play we'd been studying, but nobody was really focusing on the task. Some pupils sat on the tables to speak over a few rows and establish who was going to Marilyns, the local nightclub, that weekend.

'Are we meeting at your place after school?'

'Yeah, my brother's getting the booze in for us. He may be able to get us some fags too, if we give him the cash.'

'Oh yeah I got paid yesterday, let us know, yeah? What you gonna wear?'

'I robbed this fucking sick dress from New Look, it's all sparkly and shit. It will look so good under the lights.'

'That should grab his attention ...' The girl winked, and then they cackled like banshees.

I rolled my eyes. Every week it was the same. Excitement would mount, nobody would focus on their classes, and all you'd hear was the girls chatter about who was wearing what. The boys largely rocked up in their jeans and trainers, aiming to get pissed up. They knew the girls wouldn't be focusing on them. No, their prey was the older men. Preferably 25 plus. There was always one particularly fit man that all the popular girls would buzz around, like bees to a hive, vying for his attention, and each girl would try her best to outdo the other by wearing a stunning outfit.

Marilyn's was the club of choice for the entire high-school population, mainly because it was the only club in town. With most of the pupils living in small villages, an older sibling was usually roped in to drive into town and pick everyone up at three o'clock in the morning, then ferry everyone back to their respective homes. Not an easy feat unless you had dirt on them, and could use blackmail. When that happened, most of the pupils in the school year would rush round to each other's houses to get ready for the club right after the final bell rung, and the poor sod who had been caught by his little sister hastily getting their parents' car fixed after crashing it the night before would be stuck ferrying wads of drunk pre-teens to their homes across the Cotswolds until dawn broke.

I'd never been inside the club, partly because of my overprotective parents, but mostly because I had no friends. Fortunately, I had no desire to enter an environment that sounded like a cattle market for old men to have their pick of over-excited girls just a year or two into adolescence, clutching their WKD Blues and tripping into the toilets with their inebriated friends.

Listening to them each week was nauseating. How were these people happy? Just sitting in class gossiping about their plans to enter some building on a Friday night to destroy their livers. Didn't they want more? I'd read stories about people who were child actors, who got home-schooled in between takes and in between exotic locations. Or authors who sat writing their books in fancy apartments, and went to meet friends and have stimulating conversation, deep in the heart of London – a city I'd only seen brief snippets of on school trips, and loved reading about. These weren't ordinary lives, or lives I could necessarily achieve, but they were lives people *could* live. It largely seemed down to pot luck, and I'd drawn the short straw. It was depressing, and I'd had enough.

That afternoon, I was trying to get my group to focus on the task at hand, but nobody cared. I'd had the misfortune of being placed with two popular girls and a cool guy, and they had no interest in giving me the time of day. As I sat and did everyone's work for them, I tried to tune out the giggling of the girls as they scrolled through their flip phones, exchanged eyeshadow palettes under the desk, and texted booze requests to the older sibling who'd been forced into being designated driver and alcohol supplier for the night.

Suddenly, something inside me snapped. Why the fuck should I do everyone's work each week and listen to their bullshit? Nobody was paying attention to the classwork. Even the teacher was not so subtly texting under his desk. I decided I'd had enough. So, I got up and walked out.

I felt a thrill of adrenaline as I wandered down the corridor. Would anyone notice me? Would they call my name as I walked away? What would I say if someone asked where I was going? I could just say I was going to the toilet. But what if it was my teacher, asking why I'd just disappeared? I thought about telling him his lessons were bullshit. I completed the tasks much too quickly, and he needed to try harder to make sure all his pupils were occupied. But I knew that he'd be angry, hurt, or both, and I'd be punished regardless. So being honest wasn't an option. I settled on bluffing some excuse that I thought I was going to be sick and was going to find a toilet. Or it could be female issues. That usually shut men up.

The toilets were the only place I could really go to; simply sitting outside or leaving the building altogether would get me in more trouble, and I was still planning to go to my next class, so I wandered inside the ladies'. The usual gaggle of girls were inside, adjusting their make-up. I knew they should have been in maths, but it looked like they'd been there for most, if not all, of the last hour. Maybe they just didn't bother going to lessons at all. I briefly wondered if I should start doing the same thing.

A few of the girls looked over when I walked in, and one of them started to say, 'Oh my God, it's Four Eyes!' But today, I wasn't in the mood.

'Bite me, you bitch,' I muttered, walking into a cubicle and slamming the door. The stunned silence was absolute and, for a few blissful minutes, I didn't have to deal with inane chatter.

Then the bell rang.

CHAPTER 3

SNIFFING OUT THE FEAR

High school stretched out ahead of me, a vast chasm of monotony that I had to get through somehow, before I could escape to university in a distant city, find out what I really wanted to do, and finally live a life of my own.

My parents kept telling me to hold on; it was only when they'd gone to uni that they had really come into their own, made friends for life, and really stretched their minds. But that didn't make the waiting any easier. If anything, it made it harder, because I knew there were several years before I'd turn 18 and start applying for places.

I dreamt of going to Oxford, studying English, and becoming a professor in Victorian literature, writing academic works, and creating fictional novels in my free time. After the school library was expanded, bringing with it 16 new computers, I developed a habit of getting to school an hour before the first bell rang so I could write in silence there. I was creating a fantasy fiction aimed at young teenagers, and the daily escape to another world made the return to everyday life more bearable. There was a space in my head where I could think about what I was creating, instead of thinking about my own existence or identity.

Friday mornings brought feelings of cold dread and anxiety, because I had double PE first thing. PE was the one subject I couldn't blag my way through. It involved being popular so you got picked for all the teams, being sociable so you could play sports such as netball and hockey, and having excellent hand–eye co-ordination. My general levels of co-ordination left a lot to be desired, and so my report card for PE consistently had F grades. Fortunately, Mum didn't care about PE either, and every parents' evening, we would avoid the table where the teacher sat; neither of us needed to be told I was rubbish at sports, and we both knew I wasn't going to try harder in lessons.

That didn't give me an excuse for missing lessons, though, much as I "milked" it every month, saying I had a heavy period and couldn't possibly attend. That gave me two more precious hours to spend in the library.

Unfortunately, one Friday I had to accept that my fake bloodbath had recently ended, and so I reluctantly headed down to the changing rooms to get ready for gym. Indoor PE was the worst kind of PE, because it involved ritual humiliation in front of both the boys and the girls. Not seeming to care that we all had different levels of flexibility and co-ordination, the teacher would line us up and have us jump over various obstacles like gym-horses. Anyone who fell over was subjected to laughter from 50–60 people.

That morning, the teacher had us queue up to vault over a block of wood, not seeming to care that we would be getting very little physical exercise in this session – unless you counted the amount of jaw exercise the girls were getting as they gossiped about which clothes they wanted to rob from the shops that weekend (actually paying for your clothes was so last year).

When it was my turn, I felt a jolt of fear. I wanted to run away, run far, run fast. I realised I had no choice but to try to get over the stupid block, with an audience of 56 pupils who all thought of me as the weird, fat loner. Anything I did from this point onwards would be subject to ridicule. Trying my best to ignore the cold ripples of fear surging around in the pit of my stomach, I ran up to the block.

As I'd predicted, my poor levels of physical co-ordination meant there was no chance in hell I'd fly over the block with the grace of my Size Six peers. I thumped into the block and fell to the ground, with peals of laughter ringing in my ears. Instead of joining the queue, I ran to the changing rooms and put my uniform back on. Then I retreated to the toilets, where I stayed until the bell rang for break.

As the usual crowd of girls poured in to re-apply their make-up and gossip, I sat looking at the door of the cubicle, wishing I could stay there. What was the point in heading out to chemistry in 15 minutes, just to copy out information from the board that I'd already studied in the textbook at home, while people pointed at me and whispered? The few who hadn't been in double PE that morning were no doubt getting briefed on my humiliation at that very moment. *Fuck it*, I thought, pulling my bag up to my lap and getting a book out. I wasn't going. I'd probably get in trouble, but I didn't care.

I put earphones in and started reading. Before too long, I'd lost track of the time. Another bell rang, and I could smell food from the canteen. It was lunchtime. Shit. I'd missed two lessons. I'd better go to my afternoon classes so I didn't get into any more trouble than I was already in.

An hour later, I walked into English and took a seat by the door, so I could walk out again if I'd had enough. Ten minutes into the lesson, a pupil from my year came in and handed me a detention slip, signed by my head of year. I felt cold. How was I going to explain this to my parents?

The English lesson slid by without me noticing what was being discussed. People paired up, not bothering to include me, and I sat alone in the corner, waiting for class to be over. No doubt it would be noticed if I walked out this time, and I'd get another detention. Now I was being watched. I couldn't even escape if I got bored. Nobody cared. There was no way out. What the fuck was I meant to do?

The bell rang, and I followed my classmates to the biology room. On our way, we passed the toilets and, without thinking,

I followed a few girls who had nipped in en route to apply yet more lip gloss. I was feeling panicky, and needed to breathe. I couldn't do that in front of an audience.

Sitting down on the toilet lid, I put my feet up against the door, and breathed deeply. Then I realised something. If I kept my feet against the door, rather than on the floor, I could make it look like there was no one in there.

The thought of not having to deal with my life sent a thrill of excitement through me. I could just stay there and read for as long as I wanted. No biology. No detention. No boring gossip to listen to. No boring weekend stretching out in front of me. I could just ... stay there.

I thought about what could happen if I wasn't found. *Can I just stay here all weekend?* It felt preferable to sticking with my usual routine. I felt so empty inside that doing this felt like it would fill me up with something. I didn't know what, but the potential consequences didn't register. I just felt pure excitement at the thought of doing what I wanted for once. No more trapped feeling.

So, I double checked I had a few snacks and some water in my bag, got a book out and started reading.

My book was pretty good, and I was known to get so absorbed in reading I'd lose track of time completely ...

Suddenly I realised everything was very quiet. Was school over for the week? I had no way of telling the time, so presumed that must be the case.

Suddenly a door opened, and I could smell bleach. Shit! The cleaners. What if they found me and I got hauled home? The door to my cubicle was locked, and my feet were still up, so they couldn't tell anyone was in there, but what if they just forced it open? Well, I had no choice. I had to sit and wait. Giving myself up now would be stupid if they didn't actually find me. I had to just see what happened.

My heart was in my mouth as I listened to the cleaners open each cubicle door and douse the toilets in bleach. It got worse when they were in the cubicle next to me. I knew it wasn't long before they'd try my door. My breathing quickened, and I felt dizzy. No. I had to stop. They'd hear me if I had a panic attack. I forced myself to breathe in for five, out for five. In for five, out for ...

A cleaner thumped against my door. 'Anyone in there?'

I froze. Do nothing. Say nothing. Don't move.

More thumping, a little harder this time. A little gulp of air escaped my mouth in a squeak.

Bollocks!

Silence. Time stretched out and seemed to last forever.

Then the shoes I could see under the cubicle moved away, the door closed ... and I was plunged into pitch black as the light got turned off.

I was alone in the darkness.

Sitting motionless, I contemplated my options. If I stayed in there all weekend, I'd be starving, unable to get out, and would be in big trouble come Monday. But if I left now, I could still get found, and I wasn't quite ready to return to my life just yet. I wanted to do something to take my mind off it.

I could go up to the first-floor computer room and browse the internet for a while. And the nurse's room had some water bottles, which would help with my increasing thirst. Once I decided on a plan, I felt calmer. But the prospect of leaving the toilets still scared me. What if someone was waiting outside? What if they'd known all along I was in there, and they were just waiting to ambush me?

But at the same time, I couldn't just sit on a toilet seat for two days.

I got up and slowly opened the toilet door. So far, so good. I felt my way to the main door and gingerly pulled it open, an inch at a time. Nobody jumped out at me, so I figured I was good to go. Very quietly, I closed the door behind me and headed to the nurse's room.

The water bottles were in a massive multipack under her desk, so I grabbed one and headed up the stairs to the computer room. My footsteps echoed in the still darkness, and creeped me out. Someone would hear me immediately if they were in here ... but at least I'd hear them, too.

I opened the door to the computer room and turned the light on. It was strange to see the abandoned classroom, a few textbooks scattered across the desks. A mobile phone had been left on the teacher's table – no doubt confiscated in class and forgotten about for the weekend, much to the annoyance of whoever it belonged to. Usually a threatening room, as it signified emptiness, boredom, and bullying, the deserted space felt welcoming for the first time.

I logged on to the internet and browsed some chat rooms for a few hours. I never joined in for fear of being mocked, like I was so frequently at school. But it helped to find spaces where people my age were talking about how school sucked, how they felt lonely and sometimes got depressed. As I had no friends whatsoever at the start of high school, it was nice to feel like I wasn't the only sad loser out there. So, I just hovered in the background, looking at the conversations flow, like a ghost. Which was how I felt most of the time, anyway, because nobody paid any attention to how I might be feeling. *I may as well not exist.*

It was so quiet I felt like I was on borrowed time. How could things be so quiet? I gazed out of the window from time to time, taking in the quiet school drive which was flanked by huge oak trees. A small breeze was in the air, making some of the plants flutter. Apart from that, everything was completely still.

Before too long, I was out of water and needed the loo. I decided to head back down and go to the toilet. But as I placed my foot on the third step, I was interrupted by a deafening sound.

Alarms.

They suddenly started blaring, piercing through the silence with deafening sound. I turned around and sprinted back up the stairs, jogging into the classroom and throwing myself under the computer desk and hiding myself by placing a chair in front of me.

A few minutes went past. The alarm kept blaring, but there was no immediate change. I pulled the chair back and walked to the window. What I saw made a cold thrill of fear plummet from my chest to the pit of my stomach.

Long red flashes of light were circling the building, indicating there had been a disturbance to the security. In the distance, I could see two police cars approaching. I ran back to the computer I'd been using, switched it off and resumed my position under the desk.

Before too long, I heard voices downstairs, and the alarm got turned off. I relaxed slightly. The noise had been freaking me out more than I'd realised. Now I felt like there was no immediate danger.

Silence filled the air again, and for a few blissful seconds, I thought the police had simply deactivated the alarm system and left again. I opened my eyes, and realised I'd had my hands in front of my face. Tears were trickling through my fingers, and I was shaking. I peeked out towards the window, and could see the blue lights of the police cars. They were still here.

Suddenly, I heard a soft padding heading up the stairs, accompanied by panting. It got steadily closer, and I froze, tears falling onto my lap. Then I heard a bark. A dog? Why was there a dog here?

Its face appeared by the chair, and I backed into the corner, pressing myself against the wall. What the fuck was happening? The creature nudged the chair slightly and pushed its way in before sitting down next to me. Then a torch light shone in my face.

'Get up, girl.'

I peered up at the police officer, bewildered. Was I in trouble? I had a name, why hadn't he asked for that? Why was I simply "girl"? There was a distinct hint of disgust in his tone, as if he didn't have time for my shit. What had I done?

'Up!'

I shakily got to my feet and followed him downstairs, the dog padding along next to us. When we reached the bottom, two other officers were talking to the school caretaker, Mr Taylor. He looked at me, instant recognition flashing in his eyes.

'It's one of our pupils ...'

One of the officers drew him to one side, taking notes down on a pad. 'Yep, the parents called us ... yeah, thank you so much for coming out ...'

They turned back to us. 'I reckon you owe Mr Taylor here an apology.'

I was so scared I didn't know how to speak. Mr Taylor gave a tired half-smile. 'It doesn't matter. No harm done. I'm going to head home, if that's alright?'

The officer nodded. 'You okay to take care of this?' he said, speaking to a sour-faced woman standing next to him. She nodded grimly, and gestured for me to follow her.

I was petrified. Where was I going? Why did these police officers seem to hate me? What was going to happen now?

I got into the back of the police car parked on the school driveway, and we started moving. I was sitting behind a section of caging that separated me from the police officer in the driver's seat. Leaning over slightly to get a look at the clock on the dashboard, I realised with a jolt it was 9.03pm. I'd been missing for over six hours.

Why had I thought this was a good idea? My parents had called the police. Mr Taylor had been called out to sort the security systems. The officers had probably been looking for me. I felt ashamed. I'd caused so much trouble, and now I had to face the music. But none of that explained why I was being treated like a dog turd on the bottom of someone's shoe.

We headed onto the main road in silence. The woman driving me looked angry, and I was scared. Was I going to be thrown in a police cell?

Once we were on the dual carriageway, she spoke.

'Confess.'

'What?'

'We know you broke into the school. Why did you do it?'

Confusion swept through me. Break into the school? How could I have done that? I wouldn't have any idea how! Besides, I'd never broken the law in my life. I was a good student. I wasn't a criminal.

'I didn't, I was in the toilets the whole time!'

'Bullshit, the cleaners do the rounds every night; someone would have seen you.'

Why was she swearing at me? I felt like crying, but knew that if I did, she'd take that as a confession. I had to stay strong and argue my case.

'I was! A cleaner came in, she didn't see me ...'

'I don't believe you.'

I couldn't believe how I was being treated.

Silence again. We continued down the dual carriageway.

I recognised the route, we were going to my house. I felt cold fear sweep through me. What was I going to walk into?

A police car was parked behind my dad's Ford Galaxy. The front door was slightly open. Apart from that, everything was quiet.

When I walked through the door, my parents barely looked at me. Mum's head was in her hands. She glanced up, registered my presence, and walked upstairs, closing her bedroom door.

Dad stayed behind. 'Are you okay?' he asked. I nodded.

He had a few words with the police officer, who left with the surly-faced woman. A few minutes later, both police cars were gone.

Mum came back down. 'What were you thinking?'

'I ... I don't know.' My voice sounded hoarse. I cleared my throat. Dad went into the kitchen and came back with a glass of water. I gulped it down, and tried again. 'I guess I just wanted to be alone for a while.'

'You could have just gone to your room! Why did you bunk off school? Where have you been? Why did you break into the school?'

'I didn't!'

'That's what the police told us.'

'The police were fucking wrong!' They flinched. As a general rule, we didn't swear in the house.

'Can I go upstairs?' I asked. The words jumped out. I just wanted to hide.

I got no reply, so I just walked upstairs and got into bed fully dressed. Cleaning my teeth, getting into my pyjamas, it all felt so pointless. This wasn't a normal day. I wasn't normal. My life was a mess, and I didn't know why.

CHAPTER 4

FIELD TRIP

Being a teenager meant I was being introduced to hormones, mood swings, increased self-awareness and an even stronger desire to be part of a group, to fit in somewhere.

I felt like I was the only loner in the school until I turned 15, and Sky arrived. Sky did not fit in from the word go. In fact, she didn't even speak. An elective mute, Sky wouldn't say a single word at school, and she was seen as a freak by both classmates and teachers alike, who did not know how to deal with her silence.

But I was intrigued by her. She was different. She didn't look at me and call me names like everyone else, because she was one of the misfits.

One lunch break, I decided not to spend my time in the toilets and went to look for her. After trawling the classrooms, I found her in the art room. She was just drawing. I'd never seen anyone look so peaceful.

'Are they band logos?' I asked, sitting opposite her and opening a book, so I didn't seem too threatening. I didn't expect a reply, and I wasn't going to push her for one. I simply wanted to spend time with her.

There was silence for a while, then I heard a faint, high-pitched voice. 'Mhm.'

'Cool. What bands?'

Sky wasn't into music like the other kids in our school. She liked heavy metal: Slipknot, Nightwish. Tattoos. It was another world from the *Girl Talk* magazines, Steps and S Club I'd been brought up around. It was fascinating.

We soon become best friends, and it didn't matter that the world thought we were weird. We had each other, and that was all we needed.

Mum didn't approve of the friendship. She thought Sky was weird, and didn't want me going the same way. In classic teen rebellion style, I ignored her and continued spending time with her. Having a friend who accepted my strangeness 100 percent, embraced it even, was something I'd never had before.

We didn't have many of the same classes together, and that was okay – except for maths. I wanted so badly to be in her maths class, because being in top set for maths (like I was) meant being with Miss Peters.

Miss Peters was known throughout the school for being utterly terrifying. If her name showed up on your timetable, you knew your year would be a miserable one. You did not want to get in her bad books, because if you were caught not toeing the line, you got hauled up to the front of the class and yelled at. She would get so close, I sometimes saw flecks of spittle hit students on the face. But they didn't dare to brush them away.

I had always been quiet in class, but Miss Peters was all about class participation. I knew that if I didn't volunteer answers to my weakest subject, she would pick on me, and if I got it wrong, there'd be hell to pay.

The concept of maths classes became unbearable. The thought of being in the classroom, faced with her presence, which was like a volcano that could erupt at any second, was more than I could cope with. I would excuse myself from spending time with Sky at lunch break if I had maths afterwards, and spend the last 15 minutes in a toilet cubicle, frantically skimming over my homework answers and praying they were right. I'd find it hard to breathe, my palms would get sweaty, and I'd start hyperventilating. Nightmare scenarios would whirl around my head. Miss Peters hauled me up in front of everyone, yelled at me for getting my homework wrong, or getting an answer wrong, and everyone would be laughing while her words roared in my ears.

One day, I walked into maths and realised I'd forgotten to hand my mobile phone in at reception that morning. It was poking out of the front of my bag. We had a school rule that we couldn't have our phones on us during the day, but we could bring them with us in case we had to contact our parents outside school hours.

Most people kept their phones in their blazer pockets, texting under the table, and not caring if they got caught, but I was a goody two-shoes and always dutifully handed in my phone to the receptionist at eight o'clock each morning.

When I saw my phone in my bag, a cold fear swept over me. It was so intense I could feel it gathering under my armpits, around my collar, and I felt the hairs on the back of my neck stand up. If she caught me, I was toast. She would not allow for an explanation, excuses, any words at all – except her own, which she would roar into my ear in front of the class.

I quickly zipped up my bag, praying she hadn't seen, but luck was not with me that day. I realised I'd left my book in my bag, and opened it again ... revealing my phone right as Miss Peters walked past.

She froze. I froze. We stayed, motionless like statues, each waiting for the other to make the first move. There was no way in hell I was going to try to fight. I knew I was done for. The sweat around my collar beaded up, and I braced for impact.

'Imogen, you have your phone in class? This is unacceptable!' she shouted, and everyone turned their heads to look. One student was even openly texting as they turned around, knowing that there was no way Miss Peters would notice them now I was on the radar.

'I'm sorry, I left it in my bag,' I muttered inaudibly.

'Don't make excuses. Get up!' she said, and I shakily got to my feet. 'Give me the phone,' she said, and I obeyed.

'This is completely unacceptable. You know what the rules are, and you have ignored them so you can do what you want. Do you know where half the class are right now? In a prefect meeting. Next term, if you thought there was any chance of you becoming a prefect, it's been ruined by this complete disregard of the rules. Now, you go and hand the phone in right this instant and come straight back here!'

I stumbled out of the door, which slammed behind me. I could feel the flecks of spittle across my cheek and wiped them away, but they were soon replaced by a flood of hot tears.

My worst nightmare had been realised, and I couldn't do anything but replay the scene over and over in my head.

I had to move, because if she caught me in the corridor crying she'd just have more ammo to use against me. So, I tripped into the playground and made my way across the Tarmac. As I did, a flood of students came out of the design and technology labs. They all looked at me curiously, then mockingly, as I stumbled over to the office. I was completely humiliated. I'd been labelled as someone who had broken the rules, when I only ever tried to be a good student. That one moment of forgetfulness had resulted in more terror than I knew how to cope with.

I knew who I was – I was a good kid. Yet she'd told me I was everything but. In her eyes, I was a bad kid. Someone who needed to be punished, yelled at, humiliated. I felt shaky, and the world seemed shimmery, like I was in a dream.

I handed in the phone at reception, barely aware of what I was doing. Then I found myself gazing up at the school entrance. It loomed above me, with a strong message: Do Not Leave.

But I had to. There was no choice. My mind had shut down, not giving me any other option.

I looked back at the receptionist, who was absorbed in something on her computer. Then I walked out of the school.

There was a feeling of deep panic in the pit of my stomach, that threatened to explode out of me; what I was doing was wrong! I had to stop!

But there was another side of me in the depths of my mind, a scared little girl, cowering in the corner, trembling and crying. 'It's already gone too far, Imi,' she whispered. 'You can't go back to that classroom. You just can't.'

My conscious mind, and the scared little girl – my Mad Traveller – nodded in unison, and then she faded away.

*

I've always been scared of water. The concept of making myself float on it was beyond my comprehension. Every time I stepped into a pool, whether I was 3 or 13, resulted in a deep panic that overcame me completely.

Water was terrifying. It could drown you. Suffocate you. The feeling of water in your nose, stopping you from breathing, leaving a raw stinging sensation when you cleared it from your system. The sheer panic I felt whenever I had to go to a swimming lesson turned me into someone else. A child. Screaming for mercy.

I could paddle with armbands and floats, but that was my limit. I had one-on-one lessons with teachers who would try to subtly take the floats, or their hands, away, but I would always know when they tried, and grab them back.

Once, I had an instructor who got me paddling with armbands, then went behind me and slowly deflated them. I felt myself sinking, and grabbed on to her. But she wouldn't let me hold on. 'You can do this!' she said, as I went deeper into the water. 'Keep moving!'

But I could feel my nose reaching the water, feel the burning sensation, and know that I was going to fall unless someone caught me. The panic turned into a roaring that filled my ears, and my nose started filling with water. All I could see was water, ready to swallow me, consume me. I screamed, but that only made me sink faster.

*

My memories of what happened after I walked out of school are hazy, but some of them have returned, semi-intact. It's like I'm looking at them through a glass that distorts the images. But it's not just the objects around me that are different. The passage of time disappears ...

I know that I walked. I walked for some time. The field that I went to was on the outskirts of the village. It was cold, and my blazer was not enough to keep me warm, but there was nothing I could do about it.

The grass was slightly damp, and the rows of green I looked out at stretched on for eternity. It felt like I was no longer near civilisation. Nobody could find me. I did not want to find myself.

The Mad Traveller had climbed into her Cupboard and closed the door. She was cosy and safe. She looked smug. She didn't have to answer to anyone anymore. She was on her own, and nobody would find her.

I don't remember doing it, but I ended up drawing what I saw on the back of an exercise book. My MP3 player had run out of battery, so I must have listened to music until it went flat. I spent quite some time drawing, and it must have taken hours.

I don't know how long I spent out there. The first solid memory I do have is the flash of police car lights. They were directly behind me, and I flinched. The lights were recognisable to me, but I did not know why. "Danger," they screamed, as they went past. But they faded away into the darkness, and I was alone again. In the dark.

Dark. I didn't know why it was dark. The green had gone. I looked down. My school bag lay next to me, full of books. I felt damp. I stood up, and realised I had to urinate. I didn't know where to go, because all I could see was black grass, so I urinated into the hedge and quickly pulled my tights back up again, as if someone was watching me.

But nobody was. I was alone. Why? Why could nobody see me? Another set of lights flashed past, and I recoiled into the hedge.

The Mad Traveller nudged her Cupboard open, then slammed it shut. Once the reverberating silence echoed around inside her chamber, she opened the door again. Slowly, gently.

I looked left and saw a row of houses way off in the distance. None of them looked familiar. I looked down at my hands, and the patterns drawn on them in royal-blue fountain pen ink.

Another car went past, and the roaring sound scared me. I jumped again, and the Mad Traveller jumped too. She fell to the floor, then stood up, staring around. She was wide awake.

I felt a wetness on my cheek, and touched it. Cold tears were trickling down my face. I got up, and nearly fell over. I was not used to standing upright. I put my school bag on, and started walking towards the houses. Maybe they could give me some answers. They might help me make sense of it all. I just had to keep walking.

The lights got stronger as I kept walking, and they hurt my eyes. When the hedge ended, I could see the cars shooting past, and worried about being out on my own at night. What if one of them had a dangerous man inside who was going to kidnap me? I wanted to be at home.

I just didn't know where that was.

Nothing made sense.

The lamps outside the row of houses gave off a warm, comforting glow. They oozed a feeling of safety that I liked. I held my hand up to one of them, and the warmth was nice. I stood there, enjoying the warmth, and watched as my skin changed colour, adjusting to the temperature.

I could see further down the road, and there were more houses. I kept walking. I didn't know what else to do.

Then a car drew up next to me. I looked at it and jumped. It was a police car. Then I realised the police could help me.

One of the windows wound down, and a man looked at me. 'Imogen? Where have you been? Are you okay? Will you get in the back?'

As he said the name, I drew it out in my head. The letters danced around, then formed a word, which clicked into place. I blinked and turned to the door. Then I got in.

As we drove down the road, the woman sitting next to the man turned around. 'Are you alright?'

I didn't say anything.

'She's probably in shock,' I heard the man mutter to her. 'Let's just get her back to her home address.'

There was a crackle, and a tiny voice came through on the radio. 'Yeah, we've got her. Taking her home.'

As the roads whizzed by, I saw bigger lights and signs that seemed more familiar. Then we turned into a road, and my stomach did a funny little flop.

I'd walked out of school. I'd disappeared for several hours.

We pulled up outside my house, and I got out of the car. I felt strangely weightless, like this couldn't be real. The police walked straight through the front door without knocking, and I wondered why it wasn't locked.

Mum and Dad were sitting on the sofa waiting for me. After the police left, there was no movement from either of them for a few minutes. All I could hear was the ticking of the clock.

Dad looked exhausted. He had grey bags under his eyes. Mum looked like she'd been crying; she had a few dots of mascara on her cheeks from where it had smeared. She looked up.

'This keeps happening. You keep running away and we don't know why. We're going to get you an appointment with a psychiatrist. There's clearly something going on here.' Mum frowned slightly as she spoke.

I was silent for a few minutes. I had to see a shrink? Those were for crazy people. I wasn't crazy. I wanted to leave, so I got up.

'Sit back down!' Dad barked, making me jump. I sat on the very edge of my seat, making it clear I didn't want to be there. I felt ashamed and embarrassed, but most of all I was tired. I just wanted to sleep and forget that it had all happened.

'Look at us,' Mum said, playing with a loose string of thread on her shirt. 'Swearing. Arguing. Police cars. What's happened to us?'

'Maybe we're just a dysfunctional family,' Dad muttered. I didn't know what to say.

The silence was absolute, and I felt like I was drowning in it.

CHAPTER 5

ROAD TO NOWHERE

The armchair needed cleaning. It had stains on it. And it was falling apart. I picked at the leather while I waited for the psychiatrist to turn around from his computer screen. It was a sunny day. Beams of sunlight were forcing their way through the window, making me squint.

I just wanted to play my guitar. Dad had handed me one a few months ago, mumbling that he'd found it in the attic, and quietly left me to see if I liked it. I did. Music made me feel better. It had hurt my fingers to start with, but I'd managed to strum out a few basic chords. Once Mum was convinced I was serious about learning to play, I started lessons in the next town over. We played some basic stuff from the grade book, and old classics. My favourite was 'Zombie' by The Cranberries. It felt good to create something. Make sound that I could get lost in. Feel the grungy tones of my Ibanez through my Marshall amp. It made me feel happy.

I was just sick of seeing this psychiatrist guy, though. He would peer at me through his half-moon glasses, and scribble enthusiastic notes in a little pad he clutched in his hands, his nose and mouth twitching like a beaver. Whenever I mentioned a feeling I'd been having, he'd urge me to say more, then tell me about the other case studies he'd encountered in the past, and how much I was like them. It was remarkable, really. Such a rare condition. He was fascinated by it. I wished he'd shut the fuck up and tell me how to fix it instead of adding my notes to his intellectual wank bank.

My parents seemed satisfied that they'd done their bit by booking me in with a psychiatrist, as if he'd wave a magic wand and within a few sessions I'd stop being such a troubled child. I wished that I could confide in him, but the thought of telling him what was really going on in my head made me feel sick. I wished I could talk to someone, but I didn't know who would really understand. So I talked to no one, and thought myself completely alone.

*

When my GCSE studies were drawing to a close, and we all started revising for our exams, it felt like life was about to change. I'd been enrolled in sixth form, providing I got the grades, but Sky would be leaving. She had never really been one for academic learning, and would be getting a job instead. Part of me wished I could just quit school and go and get a job with her, but I knew I had to deal with two more years before escaping to uni.

I knew that September signalled new beginnings, but one thing would return to the way it had been for years: loneliness. I had no friends. I knew I would be sitting through lunch breaks on my own again.

Although school had generally been better when I'd been spending time with Sky, I still wasn't allowed out much. I wasn't a very sociable person anyway, and spent most of my free time reading, alone. After years of bullying and being treated like a freak, I'd embraced the label. Choosing to listen to Slipknot and Nightwish, reading *Kerrang* magazine and planning what tattoos I wanted to get helped me feel like the person I could be. Alternative. Weird, but in a good way. Part of a community of people who didn't belong in mainstream society.

I'd started seeing someone in secret. We met one afternoon on the bus home from school. He only lived a few roads down from me, so it was easy to meet up and just tell my parents I was at an after-school club. We spent time at his place most evenings after school.

I'd been listening to other people in school discuss having sex, and knew it was something I wanted to try. But when I mentioned it to him, he got much too excited at the prospect.

One afternoon, he took my clothes off without asking me if it was okay, and I found myself having sex without wanting it. I bled onto the floor, and went straight to my room when I got home. I felt broken, and curled up into a ball. People were doing things I didn't like. I didn't know how to cope. Nobody seemed to notice or even care that I was hurting so much. I wanted to get away. I had to leave. I had to go somewhere. Anywhere but my life.

*

My feet carried me down the street. I was not fully in control of the process, for my mind was not there. All I remember is the sensation of my feet on the pavement, walking at a rapid pace. Where was I going? I did not know.

The Mad Traveller was buffeted along by my movement, sat inside her Cupboard, merrily doodling away on a sketch pad. She was not too concerned about where we were going. All that mattered is that we were going. Away. Moving away.

Moving away from what? My mind waded through the grey fog that had risen to the surface and clogged up my thoughts. But wherever it looked, it drew a blank. There were no answers. No coherent thoughts. There was nothing, and that raised alarm bells in my mind.

There had to be something! I panicked internally, and stopped at a bus station. The Mad Traveller looked up briefly, then nodded to herself, returning to the sketch. A bus meant going away. Going away was good.

I was driven by a strong force to escape; a feeling that anything would be better than what I was fleeing. But what would I do? Where would I go?

The answer appeared in front of me before I had time to think. A double-decker bus pulled up to the station, headed for Stratford-upon-Avon. This felt right. I didn't know why, but it did. I was leaving for somewhere I couldn't be found. At the back of my mind, I knew that people would look for me, but I refused to coax the complete thought process out, because I knew that would mean I'd feel I had to return. And returning would be bad. Whenever I thought about slowing down, or going back, alarm bells would start blaring in my mind, and the Mad Traveller's face would get green and sweaty as if she felt queasy. No, going back was not an option. Escaping was.

I went on auto pilot and got on the bus. I climbed the stairs to the top deck, and was glad that it appeared I would be alone. I needed time to think. But think about what? I had no solid plan. All I knew was that I couldn't face clawing through the fog to come up with nothing again. So, I placed thoughts in my mind. Memories. Old memories ...

*

'You can't be friends with her!' Belle yelled at us from outside the treehouse. I looked at Sarah, and we giggled. It didn't matter if Belle was angry. We knew we were best friends. That's all that matters when you're 10 years old.

'Belle and I used to do everything together, but you're here now,' Sarah told me, and we got our books out. We closed the door of the treehouse to mute Belle's yelling, and started reading.

We were in the top set for English, and in the top one percent whenever it was exam time. I was usually number one, and she was number two. In science, she was number one, and I was number two. That's how it worked.

We used to sit in the treehouse or walk around in the fields. My mum had moved me to a village school not long after my ninth birthday, because being a part of the 40-strong class meant I didn't feel confident enough to speak up. So, I'd been moved to a smaller community where it was hoped I'd come into my own.

Every day, I was driven through tiny villages in the Cotswolds and dropped into a school in the middle of nowhere.

We were surrounded by nature all the time. Fields, bushes, flowers, trees. Break time was no longer standing in a grey playground that was clogged up with gaggles of schoolchildren making noise. Sure, there was a playground, and kids would be noisy no matter where I went, but now Sarah and I could wander into the trees and sit on log benches in the clearing. Or we would sit inside the tree house with our books and lose track of time, only being summoned in when a teacher came to look for us. But we were never told off, because they knew we'd just lost track of time. We were top pupils, and understood all of our lessons. School was easy. Life was a breeze.

At home it was noisy because of my brothers, so I would often go to Sarah's house in one of the tiny villages down the road from school. We'd sit in her massive garden reading each other gossip about S Club 7 and Steps from the latest issue of *Girl Talk* magazine, and filling in quizzes for each other. We drew posters for science projects, painted each other's nails, and played with her hamster, watching him roll around in his little ball.

I wrote stories. Whenever we went on a school trip, I would write about everything I saw. One winter, we went to a Cinderella pantomime. I was entranced by the colours in the costumes, the expressions on the actors' faces, the beauty of the dialogue and the music. When we had to submit a story about the trip, I handed a teacher my narrative. A few days later, she sat me down in an empty classroom once school was over.

'Did you write this yourself?' she asked, showing me the paper again. I nodded. Of course I had. 'Are you sure? You had no one to help you?' I frowned.

'Why would anyone help me? Dad is busy, Mum's always busy with my brothers, and Tom is autistic, so who would write it for me?' I felt upset. This was my favourite story, and I was being told it wasn't mine.

They called my parents in for a meeting. I sat in the corner of the classroom with my Pikachu toy trying not to cry as the serious conversation went on.

Then I got told I was being assigned to NAGTY.

'What the bloody hell is NAGTY?' I asked.

My parents frowned. 'Where did

you learn that expression?'

I smirked ...

One PE lesson, I hadn't been able to find my PE top, and I didn't fit in any of the spares because I was tall, so I was stuck in the class with Mike while I looked for it. After 10 minutes, I gave up and opened a book. Mike hadn't bothered starting to get changed. He didn't often bother with much, unless it was drawing pictures in all the textbooks. He liked drawing massive penises in the history books on top of all the photos of famous figures from the past. But at that moment, he was just drawing on his planner.

'Bastard thing,' he said, shaking his gel pen. No ink came out, so he shook it some more. The gel suddenly spurted out and covered his arm. 'Fuck!' he yelled, getting a paper towel to dry himself off.

I giggled, and his head snapped around. 'What the fuck are you looking at, four eyes?'

I wiped the grin off my face and assumed a deadpan expression. 'Nothing,' I replied.

'Whatever, fish lips.' I was often called fish lips or four eyes due to my large lips and glasses. Sometimes I would stretch my eyes out so they popped, going beyond the frames of my glasses, and he'd get properly freaked out. Sensing I had the capacity to do that again – and knowing he didn't have an audience to play up to – he let it drop.

'Why don't you swear, anyway?' he suddenly blurted out. I was thrown. 'What do you mean?'

'Well, you're not like the rest of us. You came in here all late from some other place, you don't use bad words, and I don't get it.'

'I just don't like using bad words.'

'Weirdo.'

'Whatever, Mike. Why don't you try to write without having a pen explode on you this time.'

'Shut up, fish lips.'

But I was reminded of how different I was. I was taller than the other kids. I had come to the school late. I didn't swear like they did. So, over the next few weeks, I listened to how the other kids swore. One afternoon, I thought I'd give it a go if the opportunity arose.

During art class, I dropped my sketch book. 'Bloody hell,' I muttered, bending to pick it up. The back of the classroom suddenly became very silent. When I straightened back up, I saw the entire back row – reserved for the miscreants – was staring at me like I'd grown a second head.

'What the fuck was that?'

'What?'

'You swore.'

'Yeah, so?'

I grinned at their stunned expressions and walked away.

Mum wouldn't have understood that explanation, and would probably have pulled me out of the school because it was a "bad influence" or something, so I didn't bother explaining this to her. 'Just saw someone say it in a film,' I said.

'Right. Well, don't do it again, it's vulgar. Anyway, NAGTY is for gifted and talented children, and they'll give you extra workshops and opportunities to see what you're really good at.'

'Can Sarah go too?' This was my response to everything.

My parents sighed. 'Why can't you enjoy this? But yes, Sarah can go if her grades are good enough.'

They were, and before too long we were spending even more time together.

My happiness was overshadowed by a growing sense that Belle was watching, ready to pounce the minute I let go of Sarah. So, I clung on to her friendship more strongly. Perhaps that's what led to the beginning of the end.

When I was 10 years old, it was time to attend middle school for three years. I felt an intense relief when I discovered I'd be attending the same school as everyone else in my year – it meant familiar faces, so it wouldn't be too overwhelming. But Sarah was restless.

She wasn't the same that summer. Her carefree happiness had disappeared. 'I just want middle school to be different, you know?' I didn't know. 'I want to meet new people, I want to do sports, I want to do cross country. It's the start of something new.'

I didn't want something new. I wanted to keep reading books in treehouses and avoiding PE class. I'd always known Sarah liked sports, but I'd just politely ignored it, in much the same way I ignored it when my great gran went on a diatribe about how bad foreign food was, and we needed to keep everything as British as possible, so there was no way in hell she'd be eating the curry my mum had made that night; it was fish and chips or nothing.

Sarah had her mind set, though. Sometimes I'd go to see her and she'd be playing netball or running laps. Once or twice, I saw Belle there.

A few weeks later, school began. I can't remember when exactly it happened, but there was a moment I knew things were starting to change.

We'd joined pools of students from other village schools, so there was a whole flood of new faces to get used to. Unlike in primary school, a set of cliques soon emerged. There were the computer geeks, the history freaks, the horse fans, and the stoners. The music nerds, the cool musicians, and then the top tier – the cool guys and the cool girls. Wheeler was one of the cool guys, who'd come from another school. Sarah had a huge crush on him. I didn't get it, myself. But I let her babble on about him after school, and during the day I'd just find somewhere to sit and read. I didn't know where Sarah was, but I just wanted her to be happy and we still had time together in the evenings, so it didn't matter.

Then chemistry classes started, and we had to pair up with the person sitting next to us. Unfortunately, I was next to Wheeler. The only good thing about it was that he was averaging a B, so I wouldn't have to do all the work for him.

He didn't want to work just yet, though. He wanted to talk. 'Sarah says she was friends with you last year.'

'I still am.'

'Yeah, I guess, but like ... it makes no sense to me, man. You ... friends with cool Sarah.'

And thus the divide appeared. I was me, and Sarah was "cool Sarah". She belonged with the cool girls. Where did I belong? I didn't know. There wasn't a group for book nerds who liked being alone. And Sarah had stopped hanging out with me in school. I soon realised she hadn't been making an effort to find me, either. She had a new group of friends who all played netball and did cross country. Like her.

Before too long, netball season started, and Sarah had practice after school. Then the other girls started whispering about me in class. In the corridors. In the toilets during lunch break. I wore trousers instead of a skirt. I didn't straighten my hair. I wore Harry Potter glasses. I was way too tall. I had no friends. I was a freak. A weirdo. A loner. I didn't even go on the school trips. Then I realised that Sarah wasn't by my side, like she had been in first school. She was in the group of cool girls, laughing at me alongside them. I'd lost her. And suddenly I had no idea who I was anymore.

*

We weren't moving. The bus had stopped. It was pitch black. I looked out of the window and saw nothing. I panicked. Jumping to my feet, I darted down the stairs. 'Please let the door be open,' I prayed. Thankfully, it was. The bus had been abandoned. We were at the end of the line.

I walked into the street, and became suddenly, acutely aware that I had no plan. What was I going to do?

Rain splashing in messy droplets onto stone slabs. Streaming down between the cracks in little rivulets.

Cigarette butts on a metal café table. Lingering smoke from a cigar recently put out in an ashtray.

Loud voices. Screams and laughter. A flash of thunder. The smell of beer. Wine. Vomit. Barking. The wind.

Cold. So cold.

Silence.

My eyes wouldn't open. Why wouldn't they open? I started hyperventilating, then realised I was holding them closed. I forced the movement, and immediately regretted it.

Water. Gushes of water. Pouring over rocks. Pitch-black skies, with slivers of moonlight reflecting onto the waves.

Two feet, positioned on the edge of a metal frame. A bridge. Freezing cold. The night air was slowly pouring in like a mist. It was so quiet.

A soft keening filled the air, and I raised my head to locate the sound. It persisted despite no obvious cause, and I waited to see if the source would reveal itself.

I was thirsty. I touched my hand to my throat, and realised it was sore. The noise had been coming from me. I was screaming on top of a bridge.

Why?

Why was I standing here? I looked down at the water again, and suddenly the raging waves took on a new, more sinister meaning. I'd been getting ready to jump. I was about to kill myself.

What had stopped me? There had been something.

Mum. Dad. Brothers. Home. School. The back garden. The English classroom. Our car, a little red Ford Fiesta. Our old car, a blue one with a dashboard covered in sparkly ladybird stickers. The primary school classroom I'd sat in at the age of eight, with a smiley teacher who made time for everyone and made us all feel special. My bedroom. My books. The smell of old pages filling my nostrils. Lying on the floor, playing with a train set my dad and brother had built. Pushing a toy car along a mat illustrated with a map of a fictional town, making very sure it stayed exactly in the middle of the path ...

These memories came tumbling over each other, like an avalanche of boulders tumbling down a mountain, and I found myself gasping for air as they returned to the surface. The Mad Traveller's eyes widened with fear, and she swam her way out of the flooded Cupboard. She hadn't been breathing. She hadn't known she wasn't conscious. She hadn't been ... there. I hadn't been there, either. So what had happened?

'Look, I'll understand if you're angry with me, or scared, and I promise I'm just taking you to the station, nowhere else. I'm a licensed taxi driver, see? I just couldn't forgive myself if I let a young girl wander the streets at night. I'm a dad myself. I'll just take you somewhere you can find your way home, alright? I'm sorry. I'm sorry ...'

The scene came into focus, and I looked at the car dashboard, where the man's hand had stayed, as if frozen in place. He had been pointing towards his taxi logo and licence, to prove he wasn't some creepy stranger driving me off to a warehouse.

So I was suddenly in the back of a taxi being driven to a police station. I felt like I should feel more alarm – such as how I'd gone from the bridge to the taxi, for example, or how any of this had happened in the first place – but I was so sleepy. I didn't care. He could drop me off anywhere he wanted, so long as I could sleep ...

I replayed his words in my head, for lack of anything better to do. 'I'm a dad myself ... dad myself ...'

Dad. I needed to call my dad. He would be worried about me. I needed my dad. I sat upright suddenly, and the driver looked at me through his mirror.

'Are you okay?'

'I need to call my dad.'

'Okay, you'll be at the station in five minutes and they'll let you make all the calls you need.'

I sat back in the seat, suddenly wide awake. I had to find my dad. I needed him.

We arrived, and I heard a click as the doors unlocked. 'Alright, good luck.'

I bolted out without saying anything else, and went inside. I don't remember what exactly I said, but I do remember being led to a police holding room to wait for him.

When the officer walked away I was left in silence again. But this time, there was a new urgency to everything running through my mind. How long had I been missing? Had I told my family anything about where I was going? Were they looking for me?

I was impatient to go home, but had no choice but to sit and wait until someone appeared. I started reading the posters just outside the cell, which advertised the hazards of drug misuse and drink driving.

Before long, I realised I needed the toilet, so I got to my feet to look for one – and felt something crinkle in my pocket. Sitting back down in confusion, I rummaged around and pulled out a piece of paper. When I read what was on the paper, I felt a strange cold mix of butterflies floating around my stomach. It was my handwriting, but I didn't remember making the notes.

Lisa, visiting uncle for weekend, he's meeting you at the station and you're spending the weekend at his place.

There was a made-up phone number next to it – probably written down in an effort to make my story look more legit in case someone found the note.

My head hurt, so I closed my eyes and drifted backwards into the mind fog. The events of the last few hours began to unfold, this time with new details ...

'Where are you going, kid?'

The bus driver's voice reverberated slightly as he spoke. Or was I imagining it? Was I just making the situation worse than it was in my head? He was just asking me a question.

'I'm just wanting a ticket to Stratford ... one way ... meeting my uncle ...' I mumbled, handing him a five-pound note. He nodded, handed me my 50p change and a paper ticket, and I scuttled up to the top deck.

I was breathing heavily, and my heart was racing, but my mind was completely blank. I was on autopilot. I was meeting my uncle. That's where I was going. That's what was happening. I was going somewhere, and when I got off ... no, no, no! The fog came back, and I stumbled through the darkness into pitch-black nothingness. The Mad Traveller tumbled to the ground, her glasses fell off and she fumbled around, blind, searching for them.

No, my uncle. I was meeting him. That's what was happening. There was no other option. I pushed the cold fog away and forced that to be my reality.

When I arrived, it was dark, and I didn't like the drunk people in the street. So I kept walking ... walking ... walking ... my feet were tired, but I kept going, because I had no choice. I had to keep moving. If I stopped, I'd be attacked. People would know I had nowhere to go. I had to look like I was going somewhere.

I felt alone. So alone. There was nothing but dark, in front of me and in my mind. I was so cold. I was hungry. I was desperately thirsty. I wanted to curl up somewhere and read my book, but I had no light to read it with. So I just kept walking, until the scary noises went away.

I didn't want to keep going. I wanted it to end. I wanted to fall ... and keep falling. But if I fell, what would happen next?

Faces appeared in my mind. My mum. My dad. My brothers. What would they do when they found out I was gone? Where were they?

My eyes snapped open.

I was bursting for the toilet, but felt too scared to move. After re-reading the note I returned my attention to the posters, and had just about memorised the number on the second one when a familiar face appeared in front of me.

'Imogen.'

Dad came inside and sat next to me. I realised I was crying. We sat in silence and hugged. His hug held a meaning I was only able to decipher eight years later, when he hugged me in the same way – the day I was saying goodbye to him in Exeter and leaving for London to try to find a new life for myself. No words had to be spoken; I knew that his hug signified he was scared, he was relieved I was okay, and he was never going to give up on me.

CHAPTER 6

THE ALLEYWAY

A year later, it was still happening.

The kissing kept going too far, the sex kept happening even though I didn't want it.

Sometimes I thought I did, but then I changed my mind and didn't know how to say it. Other times, I wouldn't be able to breathe due to his weight on top of me, so I couldn't say it. Every time, I bled, and I felt like I was bleeding inside, too.

It started to hurt whenever I went to the toilet. I would cry out, and spend hours in the bathroom, praying for the pain to go. Doctors told me I had an infection. I was told to wipe properly, as if I didn't know how to use toilet roll, and I was given so much cranberry juice I could almost feel it sloshing around in my stomach everywhere I walked.

I stopped going to his place, and he didn't bother contacting me. It was over, but other things were only just beginning.

*

My reflection looked at me from the other side of the train platform. I was wearing a blue jacket with a food stain on the front. The credit card had my mother's signature on it, but I had signed my version of the squiggle when I'd paid for the ticket, and no questions had been asked.

It's not like it mattered. It was just money. Something people had invented to facilitate the exchange of goods and services. It didn't actually mean anything. So it didn't matter that I was spending money that didn't belong to me.

What was ownership, anyway? Why were certain amounts of money allocated to certain people? It didn't seem fair to me. I'd watched the news, and heard about people who weren't given enough benefits money. People who were dying on the streets, while other people sat in luxurious mansions with piles of money they weren't using in their bank accounts.

Some argued that the rich people worked harder for their money and the poor people were just lazy and deserved everything they got, but I'd spoken to a homeless man who'd told me he'd lost his job and been evicted. His ex-wife wouldn't let him see his children once he was on the street, and he spent his time eating leftover food in McDonalds and sitting outside asking people for whatever change they could spare. He'd lost everything and had no way of getting it back, while some rich people only got their money because they had rich parents. It didn't seem fair, and so the concept of money was pointless to me. It wasn't being used properly in society anyway, people didn't care how much went to which person, so why the fuck should I pay attention to how I got money for stuff?

Besides, I needed to get away. I was going to start again in London. It would be fine. I'd just sleep in some 24-hour toilets, perhaps in a big Tesco or similar, and wash myself in the sink. I'd carry a store of food and water in my rucksack, and find a job in a café, or something. Most people didn't ask for CVs, and if they did, I'd just print one off in a nearby library. It didn't matter what the CV said. It just had to say some bullshit that would allow some employer to give me a job. They probably wouldn't check it was true. And if they did, I'd just move on and find something else.

London would be better. I could find a life for myself and be whoever I wanted to be.

*

The streets were busy. So many people. The London Eye was in the background, but when I'd tried to get near it and see if I could go on it, there was so much jostling and shouting I'd felt nauseous with anxiety.

Oxford Street was okay, but it wasn't as glamorous as I'd thought it would be. A man was spitting into a drain in one of the side streets, and people stood in groups outside the big shops, screeching and clutching takeaway coffee cups. They all had somewhere to be, a plan for the day ... and I didn't know what I should be doing. All I could think about was avoiding people, but there were people everywhere. I wanted to be alone, in a wide empty space, where I didn't have to think, but there was so much to think about and take in. I wanted to leave, but I had nowhere to go. In a city full of people, I'd never felt so alone ...

I opened my eyes. I was curled up on the grass in a small park. It was a bit wet, but it was soft. I liked the smell. It reminded me of sitting in a garden, breathing in the air just after rainfall. I would stretch out on the ground, feeling the damp soak through to my skin, and knowing that I was part of nature.

I couldn't remember how I'd got to the park. I moved my legs, and my foot touched something on the ground, which rustled. A shopping bag. It had hard things inside it. CDs. I took some out ...

Slipknot. Nightwish. System of a Down. All bands whose albums I desperately wanted, but couldn't afford. I'd just bought them. With what? I remembered the credit card. It was in my back pocket, with a long sheet of paper around it. A receipt. I froze.

'Just sign here, please,' the guy had said, and I'd copied the signature onto the dotted line. I felt a vague sense of dread in the pit of my stomach as he looked at it, but he smiled and handed me the bag.

I walked down the street, and saw a police car. I quickly turned into the next street. What if they were looking for me? I couldn't be found. I was fine. Everything was fine.

My head hurt. I was thirsty. My water had run out. I wanted more. I sat up, and found a bench to sit on. There was a train station down the road. It was starting to rain. I didn't want to get wet. So, I got up and started walking. Everything around me had a shimmery edge to it. Maybe the water was getting in my eyes ...

I could hear voices in an alleyway. They sounded angry, aggravated. I looked over and saw a gang of men jostling each other. One of them got shoved against a massive dumpster. He fell onto the floor, and the other men started kicking him. I gasped, and stopped walking. Then I realised I'd become their next target if I just stood in the middle of the street. So I crossed the road, stood under the shelter of a doorway, and kept watching. It was like watching a train wreck. I couldn't stop it, but I also couldn't stop looking. I had to see what happened. I just had to.

The men kept kicking. There was blood spattered on the floor. I winced. I'd never been good with blood. But it was so dark it almost didn't seem real. The deep shade of red was almost black. It blended in with the dirt on the floor.

Then I heard a gunshot.

Blood poured from the man's chest. I started to scream, then grabbed my throat and forced it back down. The men walked away.

In a daze, I wandered over to where the dead man lay on the ground, no longer caring if I was at risk of being discovered by his attackers. His eyes were wide open. They were gazing up at the sky. A single drop of rain ran down his cheek, making it look like he was crying. I started to cry too, and looked for a tissue to wipe my eyes.

My hand hit concrete. I jumped, confused. I was sitting on the floor outside the train station.

Leaping to my feet, I raced back to the alleyway, but it wasn't there. I must have already come this way, but I didn't recognise the streets. Had I walked past the alleyway to another train station after seeing the dead man? Or had it all been a dream?

*

'We just want to know where you've been,' Mum said, darting anxious glances at the bag full of CDs.

'Where did you get all those? Have you been shopping?' the police officer asked, taking a few of the records out and rifling through them.

I didn't talk. I couldn't. There was nothing to say.

*

Life has an almost relentless habit of rolling on, whether you want it to or not. More than anything, I wanted to take a step back, stop, try to work out what was happening, but there never seemed to be any time to. Each morning, I had to go to school, and sit in lessons until the final bell rang. Every weekend, I found myself walking into town and back with Dad and my brothers, then awkwardly standing in the kitchen so Mum would be satisfied I was "helping out" with chores.

The psychiatrist appointments were meant to be "fixing my problems", as Mum exclaimed to me one afternoon when she was feeling stressed. I understood what she meant, and knew where she was coming from. She just wanted me to get to university and have a happy life. But I got a feeling that taking care of my brothers on her own was stretching her too much to realise that I wasn't getting "fixed". I was just getting stared at in a nondescript room once a month by a man with fancy letters after his name. And so I muddled on, hoping that maybe one day my "problems" would fix themselves.

The school year slowly creaked to a halt, and summer crept in, almost lazily. The days became longer and brighter, and I could spend more time on my own, playing music.

My guitar lessons took place with the door propped open, and a cool breeze would sigh in. Time seemed to stand still when it was just me, my tutor, and my guitar. It felt like no time at all had gone by whenever he told me it was time to pack up.

One morning, he told me that the music college was holding a Rock School, and I should think about signing up. 'I think your skills are up to scratch, and it's a good way to make friends,' he told me.

The concept was simple. Spend a week with three or four other people as a temporary band, come up with a few songs, perform them on stage to an audience on the Friday evening. Simple enough, but terrifying in my mind. At school, I was the freak. The loner. The weirdo. What if I spent the week by myself, because no one wanted to be in a band with me? What if my group hated me, and made my life hell for five solid days? Worse yet, what if I got up on stage and made a fool of myself?

But the alternative was sitting in a room on my own for the week, with books my only company. My parents couldn't find a reason not to let me go, and so one Monday morning at the start of August, I found myself boarding a bus to Stratford-upon-Avon with my guitar and amp.

When I arrived, I was overcome with fear. A huge room of people spread out before me, like an ocean I was drowning in. I sat in a corner on my amp and avoided eye contact.

An hour later, my fear of sitting on my own for the week had disappeared, as I'd been put in a group with three other people. Saoirse, Ryder, and Jack were into the same sort of music as me, and the hesitant small talk soon became more comfortable after we'd stumbled our way through some songs together. When the day was over, I swapped numbers with everyone, and realised I felt weird. Sitting on the bus home, I realised what was missing. Worry. I wasn't worried. I felt lighter. Happy. These people hadn't rejected me. In fact, I was one of them.

As the week went on, we spent more and more time together outside of band practice. One afternoon, we went to meet some of Ryder and Jack's friends by the river, and I got talking to a guy named Frank. After a few hours, he told me I reminded him of his friend Jasper.

'You two should meet, you'd really hit it off,' he told me.

That night, he connected us on MSN Messenger.

'You're welcome,' he told us, sending a wink emoji before leaving the conversation.

At first, it was awkward, as we'd been thrown together without knowing much about each other, but before too long, the conversation flowed. He was eloquent, intelligent, and had a good sense of humour. I hadn't seen a photo of him, and had no idea what he looked like, but I found myself getting butterflies in my stomach whenever I thought about him.

Friday rolled around, much too soon, and I felt painful pangs in my stomach at the thought of not having a reason to keep returning to Stratford that summer. I spent the evening getting ready for the gig at Saoirse's place, and she said we could meet up later that summer. I felt hopeful that maybe I'd found somewhere I could be happy, and it was just that I hadn't been with the right people in my hometown. I wasn't actually a weirdo, I just hadn't met the right people yet.

Once we were getting ready to go onstage, I felt panicked. There would be hundreds of people watching ... but I'd be with my friends. "Friends ..." it was a word that made me feel warm inside. I wasn't used to having more than one. Suddenly, I'd picked up several. I walked out onstage, and my fear melted away.

The night was a success, and as I headed home, my phone pinged. Jasper was asking how the gig was, and if we could meet up next week. I smiled. Something was happening, and it felt good.

CHAPTER 7

THE DRESSING GOWN

I was in love. Hopelessly in love. Jasper was my world, and I was pretty sure that I meant everything to him too. It was like being wrapped up in a warm blanket, knowing that I had someone who cared unconditionally about me. Someone who checked in with me regularly, and wanted to spend time with me. I felt safe, I felt wanted, I felt like I had an identity. I was Jasper's girlfriend.

School was miserable, still, and so by the time I reached Year 12 at age 16, I had stopped wanting to go. Sky was working in a shop, so I spent my breaks between lessons alone. I felt that the longer I spent watching everyone go out and have fun, feeling like I didn't exist, the quicker I would fade away into nothingness.

I wanted to go somewhere I felt like I mattered. It wasn't sixth form, it wasn't home. So every morning I would pack up my school bag like usual, get on the bus to town, then stay on it and travel to Stratford-upon-Avon. I'd knock on Jasper's door, and he'd answer in his dressing gown. We'd head up to his room, and just lie in bed, revelling in the fact we had each other.

Jasper had ME and fibromyalgia, which made things difficult sometimes. We were a few months into our relationship, and I spent more time watching him sleep or drink caffeine than anything else. I would feel guilty if I suggested going into town, because the exercise would take it out of him for a few days.

And although he hid it, I knew he was constantly in pain due to his fibromyalgia. 'It feels like I've climbed a mountain, even though I've barely left my bed,' he told me once, wincing.

So, I spent time massaging his legs, which were frail due to the muscle wastage, and watched him smile as the pain disappeared for a while. I just wished that I could take it away forever.

I was still struggling though.

I couldn't stop thinking about the brief relationship I'd had before Jasper. It had been so secret, it had been easy to pretend it hadn't happened. At least, it used to be that way. Jasper was a virgin, and I had to admit I wasn't. The fact bothered him, as he'd wanted us to lose our virginities to each other. It made me feel ... dirty. As if I'd been tampered with, before meeting the right person.

And the more I thought about it, the more I realised ... I had been tampered with. One night, as I tossed and turned in bed, the word "RAPE" appeared in caps in my head. I tried to rub it out, but it wouldn't disappear. It had been inked into my head with permanent marker.

From then on, whenever Jasper kissed me, or we started making out, all I could think about was the pool of blood that had been left on the floor after my last encounter with ... *him*. The previous guy. The one I didn't want to give a name to.

Mum didn't know I wasn't a virgin, and so when I'd started complaining that it hurt to urinate, she thought I must simply have had a problem with my bladder. I knew that it had only happened since I'd started seeing *him*, and every time I went to the toilet, the flash of pain I got simultaneously brought about a flash of painful memory.

I'd had an operation in the summer to try to alleviate the pain, but it hadn't done anything. I felt like I'd been permanently damaged, and whenever I watched Jasper sleeping contently in bed, I'd lie next to him, curled up into a ball, wishing someone would take my pain away.

Even when the physical pain left me for a while, the emotional pain remained. Ever since it had happened the first time, I'd felt dirty. Like I no longer really mattered. Although I had Jasper now, I couldn't help but feel that I wasn't quite good enough for him. He deserved better. I was just some strange, sad girl who had been through a lot of difficult stuff and had mental health issues. Why would anyone want me? I wasn't just broken mentally, I was broken physically, too. Every time I bled on the toilet, a nagging voice in my head would remind me that I was nobody special.

Still struggling.

A few months down the line, my school noticed I was barely attending classes, and started sending voicemails to my parents' landline. I simply got through the door before my mother arrived home from the school run with my little brother and deleted them. By that point, I was planning to leave, anyway. It was just getting too difficult at home. All I got was shouting and fighting, followed by being invisible in school. I just wanted to talk to someone, but nobody seemed to care. The only safe haven I had was with Jasper.

One day something inside me broke. It was like I'd been hanging on by a thread without realising it, and that thread was fraying more and more until it finally tore in two, with barely a sound. So, I woke up and ate breakfast as usual. I got my school bag out, and I packed some extra pairs of underwear and another outfit. I threw in some basic toiletries. Then I wrote a letter to my mother. I don't remember exactly what it said – I was in too much of a trance to be fully aware of what I was doing – but I know it said I was leaving. I tucked the letter under her pillow, because I didn't want her to find it straightaway and sound the alarms. I needed time to get away. But she'd find it when she went to bed, and know that I hadn't had something bad happen to me. I'd chosen to leave, and I could look after myself. I didn't want to leave my family feeling worried about me, so it was always part of the plan to communicate with them when they contacted me, to tell them I was okay and staying with a friend. I just needed time to get away and establish a plan.

Once the letter was in its safe place, I walked to the bus stop, feeling slightly shaky. I was leaving. I wasn't going home that night. And if I could help it, I wasn't going home ever again. I got off the bus 45 minutes later in Stratford-upon-Avon, and started walking.

Jasper wasn't expecting me that day, and I knew that if I just appeared at his door, and his mother, Kate, was there, it would be a sure-fire way to get me put back on the bus home. I couldn't face going back to the life I hated. I wanted change. I wanted to be someone new. I wanted to be Jasper's girlfriend, but more than that I wanted to be someone who didn't get ignored; someone who didn't feel alone all the time. I wanted friends, I wanted space to breathe, and I wanted to live without all the shouting. I wanted my chance to find out who I really was.

I walked out to the field where Jasper and I had first kissed, and lay on the grass, looking up at the sky. It was autumn and starting to get a bit cold, but I'd be alright for a few hours. Without thinking, I texted Jasper. *I'm in Stratford, I'm not going home,* I said.

A few minutes later, he replied. *Imi, I agree you need to leave, but you can't without making a plan. Where are you?*

Outside. Chilling, I replied, then giggled. It felt so silly. Of course I had no plan. But I also knew I couldn't keep going on like I was. I'd have slept in the field if I had to. I just wanted to escape ... start again ... be someone new.

Five minutes later, he replied. *Come over. But that isn't me saying you can stay. We need to work something out.*

Half an hour later, I was lying in his bed, grass stains on my school clothes. I changed into a normal outfit. 'I can't go back now I've left,' I said.

He looked at me. 'I know. You won't be able to do this again. I'll talk to Mum.'

*

And so began the weeks of arguing with social workers and police officers ... Attending interviews at the local college so I could transfer my A Level studies over ... And applying to local housing associations in an attempt to find somewhere new to live. I couldn't stay at Jasper and Kate's house forever, that wasn't allowed.

As the weeks went by, the situation became increasingly fraught. The house was too crowded with me there. Nobody was listening to what I wanted. Everybody wanted me to go home. But I knew if I went back, I would have to face the endless bullying and the shouting. I might see *him* again, and I could end up having ... it ... happen all over again. Nobody seemed to care. I knew I had to get out.

There was a feeling deep inside me that I couldn't shake. It told me that this was my one chance to try to make a future for myself. I had to do well enough at my A Levels that I could go to university. I wouldn't do that in my hometown. I was too messed up by the memories surrounding me there.

There weren't many choices left: I'd be forced to go home, or I'd get sent to a rough shelter. But the Mad Traveller had ideas of her own and started to wreak her own special kind of havoc.

*

'Imi! Imi, where are you?'

I stayed silent. I knew Jasper was worried – I could hear the stress in his voice – but I wasn't ready to be found yet. I couldn't be found.

The Mad Traveller stood, frozen, one foot inside the Cupboard. We were both uncertain. Poised, waiting. But for what?

I heard footsteps. He was running in my direction. I had to leave. The Mad Traveller leapt into the Cupboard and slammed the door shut.

My heart was pounding like a jackhammer, but I moved as quickly as I could through the damp bushes. I just needed to be alone. I didn't know what was going on in my head and I couldn't be near him. I didn't know what he would do.

My dressing gown was wet around the edges, and covered in leaves. I furiously brushed them off, and they fell onto my feet, which were encased in slippers. I must have looked ridiculous. But then, I hadn't exactly been thinking straight when I'd run out of the house.

My thoughts came to me through a mist, slightly distorted, as if they were voices struggling to push their way through white noise on the radio. I knew they existed, and I wanted to listen, but it was so hard. Facing up to reality felt impossible and filled me with so much fear.

I let the white noise filter out. Sitting down on the grass – I no longer cared that it was wet – I let my mind consume itself with replaying what had just happened. Making sense of it wasn't going to happen right away, but the images were swirling around my brain, and I had nothing else to occupy myself with. I was alone, and it was completely silent.

The first thing I remembered was the fear. I was sitting in a lounge that was not familiar to me. The books lined up on the shelf, the candles emitting a warm glow from the coffee table, the two cats that were wandering around, faintly mewling. None of it familiar.

A man sat opposite me, gazing at me, looking troubled. I looked up at him and felt scared. Where was I? What was happening?

Eventually, he sighed, and walked out of the room. I rose to my feet and followed him out. It didn't feel right to sit in a strange room alone. What if someone came in and tried to hurt me?

The man picked up a pack of Marlboro Golds, flicked out a cigarette and stood at the back door, fiddling with the lighter. He cursed slightly as it refused to co-operate, then I saw the flame engulf the end of the pale white stick. He inhaled, sighed, and wandered out into the garden. I followed him.

He sat down on a bench, and gently patted the seat opposite. I obeyed his silent command.

'We can't go on like this. It's causing too much stress, for Kate, for me. I can't justify having you here if so much is going wrong all the time. Kate's not mad at you, and nor am I, but the stress is getting to her. It's getting to me, too, but I'm more concerned about her. And about you. Do you think your shrink had a point? I know he's a bit of a cunt, and you said he never helped, but I've done some research online, and I can't figure out what else this could be. It has to be fugue. Are you okay?'

I was hyperventilating. I didn't know who he was, or what he was talking about, but it was clear he meant me no harm – and I was just hurting him. I just couldn't remember what it was I'd done. Had I done something terrible? Had I been violent? Why was I making two people stressed and miserable? Where would I go if I couldn't stay there? *Who was I?*

The questions came thick and fast in my mind, and overloaded my brain. I couldn't breathe properly. Remembering how to inhale, exhale, inhale, exhale, was too hard. There was too much else going on.

The garden was slightly out of focus, and I felt the same. Like I wasn't quite there. I was a hologram, not quite real, but with a presence that made no sense. All I knew was that I was upsetting people, and if I was causing pain, then I had to leave.

I jumped to my feet and ran out of the garden. Through the kitchen, through the lounge and towards the front door.

Shit! I could hear the man fall over in his haste to get to me, and his urgency suddenly felt like a threat. It was a trap. He was making me feel guilty on purpose. He had me trapped there. I had to leave, fast.

The key was in the lock, and I turned it. It wouldn't budge. Clockwise, anti-clockwise. Come on! I could hear him coming towards me, and I yanked at the handle in desperation. The door opened, and I fled.

The streetlights were all that guided my way as I ran down the road. It was cold, and the dressing gown I was wearing flapped around me. Angrily, I did it up tighter as I ran, and tried my best to ignore the biting cold that nipped at my ankles.

'Imi!' I heard the now familiar voice as he tried to keep up with me, but adrenaline drove me on, and I remembered how much I loved to run when I was outside. The burning sensation in my feet and chest soon gave way to pure enjoyment, and I found that all I wanted to do was run, to fly through the night.

The streetlights faded, and I was soon in a quieter part of town. Little cottages lined the streets instead of townhouses, and I knew I was far enough away that I could slow down.

As I rounded a corner, I saw a field. A distant memory flickered in my mind, and I saw another field, from the past, where I'd sat and drawn the countryside, hidden in the bushes, while police cars sailed past me, sirens blaring. Nobody had found me then, and they wouldn't find me now.

I ducked under the gate and dived into the bushes.

*

'You were calling me Jack, Imi.'

He was smoking again. It seemed we spent most of our time in the garden doorway, with either me watching him smoke or asking to light up myself. 'You don't want to end up like me,' he said, reluctantly handing over a cigarette. It wasn't long before I was buying menthols and sitting out with him in the garden, where we polluted our lungs together in companionable silence.

'Imi? Are you still there?' His voice was hesitant, timid, and I looked up in surprise. I was upset to hear the amount of pain in his voice. He genuinely thought I'd been about to lose it again.

'I'm sorry. I just ... I don't remember.' That wasn't the complete truth, but I didn't want to admit that I couldn't remember big gaps in my immediate past.

When I tried to recall a point I'd been calling him Jack, though, I got a flicker of recognition. The name sounded familiar, but I didn't know why. I had no friends or family called Jack. The word should have been alien to me, but it wasn't. Whenever I tried to grasp on to the meaning behind this recognition, it would ripple and flicker away, like rain dropping onto a pool of water, scattering my reflection and forcing it to instantly fade.

I couldn't tell him how broken I felt, but he knew something wasn't right. 'I don't know how to fix this. I'm sorry. Maybe I should go and see the fucking shrink again. I don't know. Can we just sleep on it?'

He looked at me for a moment, his face impassive, then nodded. Putting his cigarette out in the ashtray, he got up, kissed my forehead and went inside.

*

A few days after leaving home, I scoured the internet, looking for places that could help me. A few housing associations came up, but Jasper wasn't convinced they could help a priority case. I filled in a form anyway, and was surprised to get a call just a few hours later.

A woman called Nikita was assigned to me, and she took my full story. Until that appointment with her, I'd been stuck listening to people telling me to just go home, not taking the time to understand why I felt unable to do that. But now, I was actually taken seriously. I felt hope.

After the appointment, a few weeks passed, and I was getting restless. Had everyone forgotten about me? I was increasingly aware that Kate and Jasper couldn't house me for much longer, and there was an unspoken agreement that by the time I started the local college in September to finish my A Levels, I wouldn't be living under their roof.

One afternoon, I was sitting in the garden, watching a cigarette butt let off smoke in the ashtray. Jasper was idly stroking the cat while reading a book. I was bored.

The phone rang. It was Nikita.

'We've found you a flat.'

I was speechless. Jasper looked over at me in confusion as a huge grin spread across my face.

'You have? Where?'

'It's just down the road from where you are now. You can move in next week, if you want.'

As I continued talking, Jasper worked out what was going on, and soon his grin was echoing mine. When I got off the phone, I bounced over to him.

'I did it!'

I was free to start my life. I felt ecstatic. Nothing was going to stop me now.

CHAPTER 8

OUT OF SIGHT, OUT OF MIND

I can't do this, was the only thought running through my mind. I stood in the back of a hotel restaurant kitchen, with people rushing about around me. There were many things I needed to be rushing around for, too, but I just couldn't. I'd just shut down. This was too much.

I thought about being in bed, playing *World of Warcraft* on my computer, ordering pizza, letting the gooey cheese slide down my throat ... ahh. That was better. I'd go and do that. This wasn't working. But ... how to get out?

'I'm just going out to make a quick call, it's an emergency,' I said to two colleagues who glanced over as I headed to the back door. They went back to their work, not concerned enough to probe further. I walked out of the door and kept walking, speeding up, walking faster, until I reached a taxi rank.

'Where to, love?' the guy behind the wheel asked. I gave him my address and got in, trying to steady my breathing. I had to look normal. Act normal.

'Just finished a shift?' the driver said conversationally. I nodded. 'Yeah, I'm a waitress, not ideal, but you know ...' I laughed nervously.

The guy laughed back. 'Yeah, it's a job, right? Beggars can't be choosers.'

I felt a twinge of guilt as we turned onto the dual carriageway. Yeah, it was a job, and I was running away from it. Like I'd run away from the call centre job, and the kitchen staff job, and the warehouse job ...

I felt like such a failure. Keeping a job, maintaining a routine outside of my flat felt impossible. I didn't know how to keep it going. I could only keep it up for a few weeks before that all too familiar feeling of dread would suddenly explode in the pit of my stomach like a volcano erupting. I'd get sweaty, find it hard to breathe, and my mind would start screaming like a siren: GET OUT. THIS IS TOO MUCH. RUN.

Why did I have to run? I didn't know, but life suddenly felt like too much, and the only thing I felt up to doing was hiding in my bedroom with my pizza and my computer games. It wasn't a life. I had no money, the debt was racking up, and I was gaining weight, but it was safer than dealing with the outside world. It was just too scary.

It had only become like this in the last six months, since I'd finished my A Levels. College had been fairly easy – so easy, in fact, that I'd barely attended, choosing to teach myself the syllabus from the chunky textbooks instead. I'd made a few friends, but the pressure of regularly going out with them had been too much, and once I stopped going to college, they soon lost interest.

I had seen Jasper regularly, and things had been good, at first. But when I got panicky, or started imagining that the shadows on my bedroom walls at night were real, it started to get too much for him. We'd been arguing more, and I'd become much too angry, throwing furniture around and regularly kicking him out. Then one day he'd told me he couldn't come back, because he couldn't risk the police showing up and blaming him. 'I love you, but I have to keep myself safe ... get help, Imi, and then maybe we can talk,' he told me, closing the door a final time and disappearing from my life.

So, I was alone. My family were only one town over, and even though I'd left because it was too chaotic, it still felt like I had an anchor, a home to go to if I really needed to. But then one day Dad came to visit, and on the drive back he cleared his throat awkwardly.

'So, I've got some news I need to share with you. I've been offered a new job, a better one, down in Hampshire, so I'm going to start spending the week down there, coming home at weekends, but ... long term, we're going to be moving down there. There's a three-bedroom house I'm waiting to buy, and a decent school for Harry ...'

I was silent. Three bedrooms. That meant no room for me. I had nowhere I belonged. I'd never felt that I'd had a place anywhere, anyway. Now it was being confirmed that the only place I could be, was on my own, in a darkened room in a flat. My boyfriend had left me. My family was leaving me. I was completely alone.

I got home and immediately retreated to my room. Before I loaded up *World of Warcraft*, I made a new application for Jobseekers' Allowance and housing benefit. Then I decided it would be easier to sleep, so I covered myself in my duvet and waited for dreams to replace reality.

Although I'd finished college that summer with three A grades, I'd deliberately selected universities on my application that I didn't really want to go to. I couldn't bear the thought of being without Jasper. Who was I going to be without him? I tried to picture myself in university halls, out in clubs, pubs, bars, classes, without him. I couldn't do it. It hurt too much. So, without thinking too much about the consequences, I deliberately fucked up my application, and told everyone I knew I was taking a year out to "get some money behind me".

In reality, I was too scared to move forwards. And that, in itself, made me feel ashamed. I had been given a flat all to myself so I could have space to think and plan my next step. But now I was just chickening out. I was just a waste of space. So, I retreated and pretended life wasn't happening.

Every day was the same: Apply for jobs. Sit on the bed playing *World of Warcraft*. Order pizza. Ignore the debt letters piling up in the post. Apply for a payday loan. Rub talc into my hair so it didn't look greasy.

Autumn turned into winter, and I struggled to keep my flat warm. I spent my days in the local library until I got kicked out, or wandering around shops just to feel the benefit of their central heating.

The nights were hard. Sometimes I wore five outfits, layered one on top of the other, but it still wasn't enough. I had a constant cold, and couldn't afford toilet roll to wipe my nose. Before long, I was using an odd sock every time I went to the bathroom.

I ran out of money for pizza. Instead, I would walk down to the corner shop, bundled up in my long winter coat that covered up the holes in my trousers, and count out 2p coins to pay for value loaves of bread. Sometimes I could afford jam. Other times, I had to pretend it was there.

I felt like I was living in a dream, and sometimes I wanted to just run. But where would I go? There was nowhere I could hide, no way of making it better. I had to wait until university could happen, but the months stretched ahead of me like an endless chasm.

Once a week I got the bus to the jobcentre and sat opposite my work coach, waiting for her to finish tapping on a keyboard before saying, 'No, I haven't got any job leads yet' and being shooed away.

It was hard to find a job I could stick to. There were no suitable jobs in the area, it was mainly call centre and retail work. I couldn't cope with the relentless nature of those kinds of jobs, so I just gave up. It felt easier to give up. The work coach didn't care. My family were off living a new life on the south coast. Any friends I'd made in college were off at university now, starting the next chapter. Jasper was gone.

Sometimes I wandered down to Jasper's road, just to stand at a distance and look at his house. Sometimes Kate came out and got into her car. I watched her drive away, and considered knocking at the door. He'd probably come out, thinking Kate had forgotten her keys ... I felt a funny jolt at the prospect of seeing him again. But then I remembered he didn't want to see me. I couldn't bear the thought of seeing the pain written all over his face again. Knowing that I'd hurt him. Knowing that I'd caused it, and I couldn't fix it. I'd fucked everything up.

It felt like nothing mattered anymore. I stopped caring about myself, and I ate whenever I could.

November rolled in, bitterly cold. I went down south to visit my family for a few days. I spent the evenings sleeping on the floor in the living room and woke up with a sore back. The train ride home was long, cramped, and crowded. I was almost looking forwards to getting in, getting under the duvet and going back to my routine of doing nothing. But when I walked through the door, I could hear a trickling noise coming from the kitchen. Walking to the source of the sound, I saw that my freezer had defrosted and started leaking water. The meagre food supplies I'd stockpiled were ruined. The fridge was in the same state.

I checked the electricity meter. It was £10 in debt and had shut off. I checked my bank account. Twenty-five pence. That was worrying ... I should have had my benefits in. Grateful that my phone hadn't been cut off yet, I called up the service centre, and was told, 'You're not eligible for your benefit this week as you were away from your place of residence.'

'But I was just with family for a few days, I still have bills to pay and food to buy,' I told her, panicking.

'That's just what happens if you take a holiday,' she said.

A holiday? I didn't consider sleeping on the floor for four days to be a holiday. So I had to be chained to my flat in order to get the money I needed to make ends meet?

'You can get a food box from your local church if you come to the jobcentre and fill out a form,' the advisor continued.

I thought about walking down to the jobcentre, filling out forms and then begging for food at the church. The mental image made my stomach churn.

I hung up, counted how many slices of non-mouldy bread I had left, made a note of how much I'd be able to eat each day until my next benefit allowance came in, then went to bed.

I wasn't looking forwards to Christmas. The time of year when everyone is full of cheer and spends money on nice food, gifts, and keeping warm by the fire made my own situation feel harder. I'd made some new university applications, but I was convinced they weren't going to bother replying.

I spent the day itself with my family, watching my brothers argue as I rubbed my sore back. Used to smoking cheap tobacco, and unable to do even that with my family, my head was sore – and my mood was well below rock bottom.

On Boxing Day, I checked my email for something to do, and saw I'd had an update on my university application account. A cold fear dropped to the pit of my stomach like a paperweight. What if I'd been rejected? What would I do? They could have at least waited until the festive period was over. Bastards.

I thought about ignoring it, waiting until I was back home under the safe cocoon of my bedsheets before I gave in to the inevitable pain, but the curiosity was too strong. Wincing as I opened my profile, I read the two words that would change my life: *Unconditional offer.*

My A Levels already complete, University of Exeter had decided to accept me as a student from the following September. I had a future.

February was freezing. The wind whipped around my shoulders as soon as I got out of the car. Dad had driven me down to Exeter, so I could attend an offer holder day. Despite the miserable weather, I could tell the campus was beautiful. There were trees, rows of flowers and even the occasional squirrel skirting between the bushes. There was just one downside.

The hills.

I was severely overweight and struggled with walking down the street. How was I going to get up the near vertical inclines that loomed ahead of me?

Dad started merrily walking up the first slope, and I had no choice but to follow. Halfway up, I was gasping for air and covered in sweat. At the top, I sat down on an icy bench, the freezing wind now a pleasant relief.

I spent the day sweating. After attending some talks, I followed a group of prospective students on a tour around the campus. But I couldn't keep going for more than 10 minutes. Giving up, I sat down on a bench and wiped my face with my sleeve, watching the group walk away. There was no way I'd catch up, and I didn't want to. I just sat there for the next hour, looking at the trees. It was so beautiful. I wanted to accept the offer – there was nowhere else that would compare, I was sure of it. After so many years of feeling alone, the prospect of living in this beautiful place felt like heaven.

But if I was going to navigate this campus, something had to change ...

A week later, I sat back and admired my handiwork. I was back in my flat, and I'd just built an exercise bike. It was the cheapest one I could find online, and I'd blown my benefits on it, but it would be worth it.

I switched on my laptop, got a playlist going, and sat on the bike. I was going to exercise every day and lose weight. I didn't want to go back to Exeter in September as the same sweaty mess. I had to be new and improved. A different me. A better me ...

A week away from getting on a train and travelling to Exeter, I'd dropped three dress sizes in four months. I wasn't entirely sure how I'd done it. But every time I'd wanted to eat crap, I'd just thought about the hills! I didn't want to be left behind anymore.

I'd been so lonely for as long as I could remember. Once I got to Exeter, I wanted to embrace the new life I'd been given. The only downside was that I had to carry all my belongings down to the south coast myself.

I hadn't heard from my family in a while, and I figured they were busy. That was okay. I felt like I could do it on my own. But before I left, I knew I'd have to get rid of some of my stuff.

Gritting my teeth, I thrust open my wardrobe doors and started chucking stuff into large plastic containers. I'd leave them outside the apartment block, on the lawn. If people wanted the stuff, they could come and get it. I had no time to sell it.

Three hours later, I looked out of the window. The boxes sat lined up on the grass, and I could see people approaching curiously. Some of my favourite books were in those boxes. I turned away and sat on the bed.

The flat was empty. All that remained was a few suitcases in the other room. My bed, once a safe cocoon where I could hide from the world, was now almost stripped bare. It was nearly time to go. I felt a strange lurch in my stomach. Was I ready? Could I really do this? Couldn't I just hide again, instead?

But as I looked at my new, smaller jeans on the floor, I realised that I could. I just had to believe in myself. The months that I'd spent on the exercise bike, or sitting on my bed, watching films and chewing gum to stave off hunger pangs, had paid off. I'd believed in what I couldn't see. I didn't know what the weight loss would look like, or how long it would take, but I'd believed in it, and it had happened. Now I just had to believe in my future, however it was going to materialise.

'I've got it, I've got it!' the man said, pulling the suitcase on board. I'd tried to haul both of my bags onto the carriage once the train had arrived, but the bigger one had slipped between the tracks and I wasn't able to get it back up.

I thanked him and pushed my bags into the luggage hold. A wave of panic washed over me. What if somebody stole my stuff? I pictured walking to campus without any clothes, books, or toiletries. I peeked down into the carriage. So many people ... yep, I was definitely staying with my luggage.

An hour later, I regretted my decision. People were constantly squeezing past me to go to the toilet or the buffet car, and the journey was rickety and uncomfortable. I half stood, half sat on my suitcase, listening to music and browsing social media feeds on my phone. I was bored, but I was getting away. With every minute that went by, the high-speed train was taking me further and further away from home, from everything I knew. And that was exciting.

I finally felt free. But freedom was also scary. I started thinking about all the things that could go wrong. What if nobody liked me? What if people thought I was a fat loser and rejected me? What if I couldn't handle the work? What if I flunked out?

The train stopped at Bristol Temple Meads. I thought about what would happen if I got off the train there. Left my bags behind. Wandered the streets. Slept in a public toilet. Got a job in a shop somewhere. Maybe that would be easier than facing uni.

I got up without thinking, and bumped into a woman who was hurrying off with her kids. She looked stressed. I realised I was being stupid.

Everyone had problems. That woman could be struggling to manage her noisy kids. Maybe she didn't have much money. She certainly didn't look happy. I had a bright future ahead of me. What the hell was I playing at?

I sat back down and watched the city streets turn into green fields as the train sped on. I was okay. I could do it.

My room at uni was small, but cosy. The window revealed a view of an identical tower block of student flats. I was the first one to arrive. One of the student ambassadors had helped me lug my suitcase up, and told me I should definitely head down to the pub for a quiz that night. 'It's a great way to meet people,' he told me, flashing me a grin on his way out.

I smiled back, awkwardly, a few seconds too late. He'd already left. I cringed, then realised there wasn't anything to cringe at. He wouldn't have seen anything. It was fine. I took a deep breath, opened the window and flopped down onto the bed.

Suddenly, I was crying. I didn't know why. I just was. *Why am I such a baby*, I thought, marching to the bathroom and furiously wiping my face with loo roll. The sharp movement stung, and the pain distracted me. Then I heard voices in the corridor.

I silently swung my bedroom door closed until there was just a small gap, and peered through. A skinny blonde girl was entering the room opposite, flanked by her parents. She had so much stuff ... the ambassadors were hauling bag after bag into the room.

'What the fuck, there isn't even a coffee machine in here,' I heard her complain after flouncing into the kitchen. I quietly clicked my door all the way closed.

This girl looked exactly like the ones at school. The girls who wore see-through tights and lip gloss and wore Size Tiny outfits. I was confident she would turn up her nose the moment she saw me. And I had to live opposite her for an entire year.

I opened my laptop and looked for events I could go to which didn't sound terrifying. Walking into a pub on my own and trying to make conversation with strangers was definitely out. But a group trip to the big Tesco could work. I did need groceries. I tentatively bookmarked the event, then started unpacking ...

I stood hesitantly at the campus bus stop. Nobody was there. Maybe the whole trip was fake. Or it had been cancelled, and nobody had told me. Just typical! But then a few people emerged from a footpath, and one of them was holding a sign which read "Tesco trip". Okay, I was definitely in the right place. Could I go over there and talk to them? What would I even say? No. Sod it. I was staying right–

'Hey, are you going on the Tesco trip?' a voice piped up. I turned around to see a short brown-haired girl standing in front of me.

'Uh yeah, I am,' I mumbled, clearing my throat.

'Cool. I'm Hayley. Where are you staying?'

'Over in Birks. You?'

'Same! I'm in one of the townhouses. Are you going to the pub quiz tonight?'

'I'm not sure yet ...'

'It should be good, I heard that place plays a lot of old school rock.'

'Oh, sweet. Maybe I'll come.'

We smiled at each other. Suddenly, I didn't feel quite so scared anymore.

CHAPTER 9

'WE THINK YOU'RE AWESOME'

'Can you pick me up? I know you're probably working, but I wouldn't ask unless it was an emergency.'

'Yeah, alright. Whereabouts are you? That'll be five quid,' my housemate Chris teased.

I'd walked out of my lecture as I was feeling rough. Getting the bus back home seemed impossible, but I knew Chris would have my back.

I was in my second year of uni, after a whirlwind 12 months which had involved a whole myriad of experiences. From my first night at the pub quiz with a group of new faces, who were much friendlier than my anxiety had let me believe they would be, to six months later, when Hayley had asked me if I wanted to live with her and some mutual friends the next year.

Now I was living in a house with three of my closest friends, and my days were spent hanging out with them, going over to my other group of friends on the other side of the city, or working on my student paper. Within a few months, I'd been promoted to News Editor, and now I managed a team of writers, keeping an eye on the goings-on in the sleepy city of Exeter.

I'd kept losing weight, and felt happier more often than sad every day. Some days, I felt so anchored to the present that I didn't even think about the past. Uni had made me realise that, although I had been an unpopular loner at school, that wasn't going to be the case forever. I had made tons of friends, there was always someone to hang out with, or something to do. I knew exactly who I was for the first time in my life. More importantly, I wasn't attached to anyone in order to know who I was: journalist, classics and English student, into running, gaming, and pub crawls. Looking back at old photos of myself made me feel like I was looking at a different person.

Each morning, I woke up while it was still dark, and wandered down to the quay, headphones in, blaring upbeat dance music. I'd quicken my pace, until I was jogging, then running, the wind making my ponytail whip crazily around and slap my neck, the crisp, cool air soothing on my skin. I did laps of the path around the river, watching the sun rise in the distance, before jogging back home and jumping in the shower.

My second-year lectures were more difficult, particularly the classics ones. I was at a disadvantage as I'd never studied Latin or Greek, and the strange languages looked like gibberish on the whiteboards and projectors. One afternoon, the guy next to me glanced over as I was frowning at a particularly confusing section of ancient Greek script and laughed.

'I take it you didn't study Greek either?'

'No way. This makes no sense to me.'

'Haha. I only did Latin.'

'That's better than me ...'

We got to our feet and started packing. 'Where are you off to now?' he asked.

'I have a gap before ancient civilisations, actually.'

'Oh, no way. Same. Do you want to get a coffee? I'm Joel, by the way.'

And so began the weekly Costa sessions, where we'd sit with our lattes and giggle over ancient texts, share our mutual love of rock and metal music, and ... were we flirting? I wasn't sure; all I knew was that my stomach turned to mush whenever I looked at him.

I told him about my past, and he understood. 'I've had some mental health issues myself,' he told me, and the moment the words left his mouth, it felt like a weight had been lifted. I didn't have to hide.

I had become very good at hiding. To all of my student reporters, I was the fun, alternative girl, full of ideas and fun competitions, always keen to help out and offer words of kindness. At home, behind closed doors, my housemates saw a very different side. After all the nights I'd spent tossing and turning, reliving flashbacks of painful nights with *him*, my nightmares had leaked into my days.

Rocking back and forth in the corner of my student room, I hit my head repeatedly, trying to get rid of the swirling images, and the sounds of his grunts as he raped me. But instead of going away, the sounds became amplified, as if someone was forcing me to twist the volume dial, higher and higher, until my eardrums were bleeding, my head was burning, and my throat was hurting.

I coughed, and it tasted metallic. Why was my throat so dry and sore? With a jolt, I realised I'd been screaming. Although a slight ringing remained in my ears, the volume dial was slowly turning back down, until there was silence.

As I tuned back into my surroundings, I heard a distant knocking sound. Was someone at the front door? I listened more intently, then realised someone was hammering on my bedroom door. The memory flooded back to me, and I recalled hastily forcing the door closed, locking myself in so nobody had to witness my pain. I could sense something was happening, and I didn't want my friends to have to deal with it. But, instead of keeping it contained, the sound had alarmed them, and being unable to check whether I was safe had only made things worse.

Every time something like that happened, the house was quieter than usual for a few days. I knew I was freaking them all out, much as they wanted to be there for me. My experiences were so far beyond their own, they had no idea how to help. Sometimes I caught them darting worried looks at each other when I left the room to go to the bathroom. Sometimes we just sat together in silence, none of us knowing what to say.

Hayley and I were watching TV one evening when she turned to me and said quietly, 'We've decided to get first aid training, Chris and I ...'

'What? Why?'

'Well, we just want to know how to look after you, in case, you know, something happens again.'

I was silent. I didn't know what to say. I was simultaneously touched they would do such a thing for me, and embarrassed that they had to resort to such measures because I was such a liability.

*

'Why is *he* still here?' Hayley hissed to Chris from the kitchen, eyes wide as saucers. She probably thought we couldn't hear her. But we could, and, try as we might, we couldn't stop ourselves bursting into childish sniggers.

Yes, Joel had come over the night before. We'd watched a movie, it had become late, I told him not to walk across the city at that time, and ... well, one thing had led to another.

He'd been very careful to say he didn't want to put a label on our relationship. But I had a great time with Joel; he helped me with all the classics work I didn't understand, and the sex was hot, but his mental health issues sometimes disturbed me. Even though he understood my issues, and wouldn't bat an eyelid when I was seeing things – choosing instead to hold me until it passed – I didn't like the way he got sometimes.

He had anger problems, and had admitted he'd broken into his ex's house when she'd "crossed" him. Growing up in rough surroundings, he'd been granted a scholarship to a posh school, and had climbed up the social ladder. But sometimes his posh accent would slip, and I'd see the angry young man underneath.

I was finally losing weight, and he wanted to keep me on track. He would encourage me to go out on runs with him, even when I was too tired, but I told myself he was just looking out for me. What really annoyed me was when he rationed out my snacks. Hiding a bag of Skittles somewhere, he'd pour out 10 of the sweets into a bowl before handing them over to me. Did he think I couldn't control myself? Why did I have to be treated like a kid? I frowned, but I didn't say anything, because I was scared.

If I didn't have him to hang around with between lectures, I'd just be sitting on my own like a sad loser. And I'd done enough of that in school.

Being with Joel was mostly fun, despite the behaviour that left me feeling uncomfortable sometimes. He had a great sense of humour, and knew all the best places to go out. But sometimes, when he got angry, it scared me. He'd knock things over, mutter threats that made me shiver, and there was a fearsome glint in his eyes that I couldn't get out of my mind. I kept replaying mental images of him breaking into his ex's house, and wondered if that violent side would come out again, should we part ways.

One night, I was waiting for Joel to come over. It was getting late, and I was concerned. Checking the time, I knew that his social event on campus had finished two hours ago. Sitting twiddling my thumbs wasn't my style, so after a few minutes of deliberating, I called him to see what was going on.

'I'm just on campus still.'

'Why, what's going on?'

'Well, I was following these girls to see where they were going.'

My stomach did a funny jolt. 'Why were you following them?'

'Well, they looked interesting.'

'Okay ... what are you doing now?'

'I'm just behind a bush, watching them. They're just talking now, in a group. I've got my knife out.'

'And why is your knife out?'

'I ... I don't know. Should I leave? I can't leave.'

'Do you want me to come and get you?'

What the hell was I saying? Why wasn't I on the phone to the police?

I headed out into the night. It was November, and the air was crisp and chilly. I shivered and quickened my pace.

Once I'd climbed the main hill to campus, I saw Joel on the floor by a bush, playing with the knife in his hands.

'How are you doing? You want to come back with me?' I asked, mildly. A million alarm bells were going off in my head. *What if he attacks me? What if he attacks my housemates?*

I'd seen that look in my brother's eyes. It was wild, tortured, confused. He didn't mean to do harm, and if any harm was to be done, it would only be to himself. I didn't want to wake up the next day and find out he'd topped himself in his room. I shushed the internal agonising. He needed to know that at least one person in the world cared about him.

Joel tentatively got to his feet and followed me. We walked in silence, and when we reached my front door, I turned to him.

'Are you going to put the knife away?'

He nodded and put it in his bag.

When he was safely in bed, I locked us both into my bedroom. I put the key inside my underwear and got into bed next to him. I just wanted to be sure that if he tried anything, my friends wouldn't get hurt.

After he left the next morning, I had to pinch myself as a reminder that I was awake. The images playing in my mind from the night before felt just like scenes from a movie. Make-believe. What had I been thinking? How could I have let him stay? I sat agonising for a while, then went for a walk to clear my head.

I considered telling the police about what had happened. I was worried that he'd do it to someone else. But part of me was convinced I could help him get better, and another part was simply too scared to do anything that could lead to him wanting revenge.

In many ways, Joel and I helped each other through our worst patches, simply by observing what was happening without judgement. I'd have been there for him unconditionally, and would probably still have him in my life now, if he hadn't betrayed me ...

One afternoon, I was lounging around at his place, while he was on his way out. As the door clicked shut, I heard a bleep on his laptop, which he'd left switched on and unlocked.

Much as I wanted to respect his privacy, curiosity got the better of me after a few minutes and I scuttled over to the desk. I felt bad about what I was doing, but I still felt paranoid after the knife incident. I didn't feel like I could trust him anymore.

Opening the email, my heart dropped into my stomach and a cold sweat broke out on my back.

Hey sexy. Enjoyed those last pics, looking good.

It was in reply to Joel's message: *Just so we're on the same page, your hubby is fine to watch us, but not while we're fucking. It has to be on the video afterwards.*

The email string was entitled *Young stud looking for MILF.*

I scrolled down through his messages. There were four other women, all married, in their forties, who wanted to have sex with him on camera and show the footage to their husbands. They'd exchanged photos. I was greeted with the sight of multiple naked housewives, followed by photos of Joel clutching his erect penis. Feeling sick, I recognised a rucksack of mine in the background in the pictures.

I'd seen enough. I slammed the laptop lid shut. How was I going to get back at him? Revenge was childish, but it would make me feel good ...

I had Joel's flat key on me, as he'd asked me to let him in later. I smiled, left the key on his bedside table, and walked out of the flat. I then sauntered over to my friend's house, sat down with a stiff drink and watched a movie with her.

A mutual friend said Joel was stuck outside his building for three hours, trying to get someone to let him in. He never contacted me to find out why I'd left. I never got any apology or words of explanation. Maybe he wasn't sorry. Maybe he couldn't explain. Maybe he simply didn't care.

'I never liked him anyway.'

Chris was sitting opposite me on my bed.

'Why are people always hurting me?' I said, blowing my nose in between hiccups and sobs.

'I don't know, but we like you, and we won't ever hurt you,' Chris said, referencing everyone in the house. 'We think you're awesome. You don't need this guy. You've got so much going for you. You're funny, alternative, clever, kind, and you do all this extra shit on top of your degree work, so you'll just be hired as a journalist straight out of uni. All I've done this week is play Xbox in my underwear.'

I smiled. I was so glad I had friends like him. It had been hard at school, feeling like the odd one out, but in this safe haven, surrounded by people who genuinely cared, I felt like I had somewhere I belonged.

CHAPTER 10

DROP ROLLING INTO DARKNESS

Summers during my time at university were always hard, but one summer was harder than the others.

The stress I'd been carrying without properly acknowledging it for years had begun to manifest as stress-induced seizures. The only advice doctors had was to see a therapist. One of them even suggested yoga, as if doing some stretches on a mat would get rid of all my problems.

Looking back, I shouldn't have been so dismissive. I know that alternative therapies can and do work, but I was just so scared every time a seizure happened that I wanted something I knew would *definitely* work. Even if it meant taking medication for the rest of my life.

I'd seen therapists. Well, they were called mental health mentors at uni. And the most mine did was check I wasn't having a meltdown over my workload, then arrange for me to have extensions on assignments if I needed them. There was a long waiting list to get a counsellor on campus, and I couldn't afford private therapy.

So, I muddled through university, slowly getting worse and trying to ignore it, until one day I found myself on the floor at home, foaming at the mouth, with Hayley and Chris freaking out on the phone to the emergency services.

Several trips to the hospital followed, but when it was determined the seizures were stress-induced, nothing really happened. I figured that I'd just have to deal with it on my own. My second year of university finished, I went to my hometown – Mum had moved back after separating from Dad – and prayed I wouldn't be struck down by a seizure when I was out in public.

Except, of course, that's exactly what happened.

One afternoon in August, I was taking my daily walk into town when my vision took on a shimmery tint. I felt mildly high, like I'd been smoking weed. I felt a strange urge to giggle, and my right arm started twitching. Even though I felt "away with the fairies", there was an undercurrent of panic pulsating through me. I had to get to safety.

I made it across the road and onto a bench. I tried to focus on my phone screen, but I could tell I was losing control of my body. I started shaking more violently. I considered calling someone, then realised I had no one to call. The street was empty; I was in a ghost town.

I stumbled towards the GP surgery. I knew that if I'd be in the best possible place if I collapsed there. But that's the last thing I remembered until my GP touched my shoulder. I jumped.

'I've been saying your name a few times now. Are you still with us?'

I nodded.

'Redditch hospital are going to take you in for the night. They've got a bed for you, and they're going to run some tests to get to the bottom of this.'

I texted Mum, and she sped to the surgery so she could drive me to Redditch.

The hospital was busy. Chaotic. We headed to the Accident and Emergency department, which was packed. I checked in and was told to take a seat in the waiting area. I was confused; the doctor had told me there'd be a bed waiting for me. By this point, my thought processes were severely impaired. The concept of a bed floated into my head, then drifted away. All I could do was sit down.

I sat there for two hours. Nobody came to offer me a bed. Nobody offered to run tests. The shaking got worse. Nobody looked at me twice.

When it got to eleven o'clock at night, I realised nobody was going to see me. There wasn't a bed available. There wasn't anything available for me. Mum had left to see a friend, and I knew there was no way I'd be able to get hold of her. There was nothing available for me.

So I left.

I didn't know what was running through my mind apart from a belief that I could walk the entire distance home. I felt the overwhelming need to escape, combined with intense despair. Nobody had seemed to care how ill I was. Nobody had stayed with me or spent very long checking I was okay.

I had spent so much of my life alone in my room, but now I was alone in a strange place and I felt abandoned. That despair drove me to disconnect from the pain of my reality.

I headed to the bus station in the hope I could at least get a ride to the town centre. The bus shelters were deserted. The buses had stopped running for the night. The place was dead.

I kept walking. I got to town on foot.

My phone battery was on 50 percent. I reached the outskirts of Redditch. A roundabout loomed ahead. The occasional car sped over it, into the night. A chill swept through me, making the hair on the back of my neck stand up. I had a vague idea of how insane it was to walk along a dual carriageway at night, but I had no choice.

My phone battery was on 30 percent. Nobody cared where I was, or whether I was safe. I wasn't even worth medical care. I was on my own. All I could do was keep walking.

Redditch is 19 miles away from Evesham. I knew I wouldn't be able to walk that far by dawn, but I'd get close enough to a village to catch the first bus home. I considered finding somewhere to sleep, but decided not to risk it. I'd heard enough horror stories about people being mugged in their sleep. I'd pulled all-nighters before. I could do it again. Keep moving. Keep going.

I headed towards the roundabout, intending to follow the road signs home. Fifteen percent phone battery left. Pitch-black dual carriageway. Walking through the bushes, staying away from the traffic. Not wanting to be seen – I was an easy target.

I got seen.

The sports car pulled into the lay-by just ahead of me. I considered turning back. Finding somewhere to hide. Waiting until the person gave up and drove away. I realised there was no point. I had to keep going.

So I walked closer and closer to the car.

'Hey! Are you okay?'

'Yeah, yeah, fine,' I said, trying to sound relaxed.

'What are you doing here in the middle of the night? It's not safe, especially for a young woman ...'

'Just been on a night out, making my way home, you know ...' I laughed. It sounded false. Hoarse. Desperate. He could tell.

'Get in the car, I'll give you a lift home. Where do you live?'

'It's fine, honest.'

'Get in the car.'

Something in his tone of voice told me I'd be foolish to disobey.

I got in.

He powered up the engine, and we sped away.

*

A LETTER TO THE MAN WHO TRIED TO ABDUCT ME

It's been almost half a decade since we met, though I'm sure you remember our encounter. It was an unseasonably cold night in June 2013. You pulled in a few metres ahead of me in your sports car. For some reason, you were wearing shades at three o'clock in the morning. You waited for me to walk up to you. You knew I had no choice. I could have run, but where to? The road was deserted, and you would have caught up with me easily. You knew this, and so you smiled as I approached you. That smile sent shivers down my spine.

You saw me smile; probably presumed I was drunk. You told me to get into the car. I told you no, but you took off your sunglasses, and the look in your eyes told me it would be foolish to disobey. Your eyes were lifeless. It was the emotional detachment of a man who had done this before ...

Perhaps I was just another in a long line of victims. I heard the click of the car doors as you locked them. You expected that tiny sound to instil an enormous dose of fear. It did. But you would never have suspected that I wasn't so scared to just give in and accept my fate.

I felt a numb sickness churning around the depths of my stomach. Beads of sweat were forming around my hairline. I sat, frozen, in the corner of the seat, as far away from him as possible. He sat, staring straight ahead, a slight smile touching his lips.

I knew I had to get out. But I didn't know how. We were speeding down the dual carriageway at 90mph. Jumping out of the car now would be suicide.

After a while, we reached a roundabout. He slowed down, then began heading around it.

As you drove down the road, I made sure I analysed the door and worked out what I would need to do, if I got an opportunity to escape. You told me you would drive me to my village. I wasn't foolish enough to believe you, but when you turned off at the roundabout, telling me we were taking the scenic route, I still felt fear. I realised then that I'd been holding on to a scrap of hope that you would stay true to your word.

You were watching me out of the corner of your eye. I imagine you were anticipating tears, confusion, anger. You had probably seen it all, on the other occasions you had abducted young women. How did you feel, when you saw that I registered no emotion? Were you disappointed? Your eyes darted away, and I seized my chance. Had you ever experienced somebody try to escape from you? I knew I wasn't your first victim, but I wasn't prepared to be yet another crime statistic.

The alarm bells had been ringing from the moment his car had pulled up ahead of me, but now they were deafening me. Now. Get out now. *Get out. Now.*

It's interesting how the mind blocks out memories that you can't process. Now that I've had time to heal, I can look back and remember exactly what I did. At the time, it was a blurry haze of movement. Now, though, I recall everything with perfect clarity.

I gave nothing away. I stayed in the exact same position I'd maintained since getting in the car. He kept driving.

Out of the corner of my eye, I saw the lock on the car door. I knew how it worked – lift up the latch, pull on the handle.

I waited for my moment.

It didn't take long.

The car began to slow down. I made my move.

Lift, pull, yank, push, drop.

I sometimes wonder what went through your mind as I threw myself into you, reached over to your door, pressed the button to reverse the lock, then threw myself out of your car. I have only recently been able to remember all of my actions – my mind blocked the memory for over two years. All I remember is falling. What were you shouting, as your car sped off into the distance? To my surprise, you did not sound angry – just confused. Perhaps it was beyond your comprehension. It was certainly beyond mine.

The Mad Traveller was free falling. Her Cupboard had disappeared. The ground opened up beneath her, and she lost her balance, stumbled, and dropped into a chasm of blackness. She tried to grab on to something, anything, but she couldn't see, she couldn't hear, she couldn't feel anything but a roaring sensation that permeated every fibre of her being.

I could hear the man's voice calling after me. The car kept moving. It sped away into the night.

I was falling. Over and over. I couldn't stop.

I rode with the force I'd generated, throwing myself out of the car.

I could feel bruises forming. I prayed I didn't break anything on my way down.

I stopped.

Silence.

I wish I could make you feel the fear that tore through me that night. I wish I could make you feel the cold that I endured, as I waited by the side of a village road for the first bus home. Most of all, though, I wish I could put you in my shoes, the day I returned to that roundabout, a year later, to find out where you would have taken me. I wish you could see that abandoned barn in the way I was forced to see it, that cold autumn morning. I hope that my actions that night forced you to rethink the way you live your life. Because now I know that they saved mine.

I was in a hedge. I took a few deep breaths, then slowly sat up. I stretched. Nothing was broken. I hurt, but it wasn't anything too serious.

I got up. I was still on autopilot. I'd escaped the immediate danger, but he could still come back looking for me. I couldn't let myself feel. If I let that happen, I knew the pain would be so intense and raw, I would be utterly incapacitated.

I had to keep moving.

Before too long, I was back at the roundabout. I turned into Salford Priors, and walked through the village. It was pitch black. Silent. A few street lights were on in the far distance. I headed towards them.

There was a bus station nearby. I checked the times. There was a bus heading to Evesham in a few hours. I just had to hold on until then.

I looked for somewhere to sleep. There was no other option. My phone was dead and I could barely keep my eyes open. I wandered down the pitch-black country lane, flinching whenever a car raced past.

A few minutes went by, and I could feel vibrations in my throat. Confusion swept through me like a dull ache until I realised I was part-humming, part-singing.

Kumbaya, my Lord, kumbaya

Kumbaya, my Lord, kumbaya

Kumbaya, my Lord, kumbaya

Oh, Lord, kumbaya.

The last time I'd sung that song was in primary school aged 10. I had stood in the back of assembly, holding a battered hymn book, reciting the lyrics along with everyone else. It was the only hymn I liked, because it had a comforting rhythm to it. I stood in the assembly hall and let the words wash over me.

The words came back to me then, and lulled me into a calm enough state that I could function. My deep subconscious knew that if I didn't soothe myself, I would do something stupid. I didn't know what, until a mental image of myself crawling into the hedge that lined the country lane came to me. I watched as my mind played out a scenario where I fell into the undergrowth, wandered into a field, and kept walking until I found somewhere remote enough that I would not be found. Somewhere I could curl up and wait ... until I stopped breathing.

The thought was comforting, and that scared me. The intense loneliness I'd experienced, the illness, and the trauma I was living in that moment, had all sent my mind to a very dark place.

The Mad Traveller was lying at the bottom of the chasm. She twitched slightly, trying to get up, but she couldn't. Something had broken, and she'd given up. She slowly raised her head towards the tiny pinprick of light miles above her, then fainted.

I sat down outside an abandoned farmhouse. The floor was probably dirty, but I was past caring. I watched one of the loose doors flap in the wind, and slowly realised I had to urinate. There was nobody around to see me piss like an animal, so I got up, pulled my trousers down and squatted over a puddle.

The urine trickled down a mud path and into the neighbouring field. Part of it splashed my shoe. I didn't care. I got dressed again and sat next to the flapping door.

It was cold. As my mind increasingly re-associated itself with my body and sense of self, that was the first thing I could feel. I looked down. I was only wearing a thin jacket. I desperately wished I had another layer on that I could cover myself with. It was pitch black, and I guessed it must be three or four o'clock in the morning by that point. There were still a few hours until dawn, and I had to wait them out.

I lay down on my side, pulled my arms up into my sleeves, wrapped the sleeves around my torso and hugged myself inside my jacket. Then I closed my eyes and fell into a half sleep.

*

The light woke me. It was a gentle light, contrasted by the artificial glow of the street lamp a few feet down the road. I opened my eyes, and suddenly remembered where I was. All the memories of the past 12 hours swept through me like a flood, and I refused to delve too far into the pain. Instead, I focused on the hope that now, my waking time could be spent getting to a place of safety – not living through a hell I could barely comprehend.

I got up and walked to the bus shelter. Thankfully, it was abandoned – I had no idea how I would explain my appearance to a villager who may arrive to catch the first journey into town. I straightened my hair and clothes as best I could, and composed myself.

Just a few minutes later, a bus arrived. I briefly struggled to remember what the etiquette was – oh, money. I needed money – before clambering onboard and throwing a handful of coins at the driver. I took a seat near the back and rejoiced in the warmth that greeted me. The engine started up, and I was on my way home.

CHAPTER 11

A LIFE ... OF SORTS

My final year of university was a blur of studying and sleeping at strange hours; the stress was immense. By some miracle, I managed to graduate with the grades I wanted, but once I left campus for the last time, my degree certificate in my bag, I wondered what life held for me.

I'd lived in this tiny, perfect bubble of perfection in Exeter, where I'd felt like I knew who I was. Once I left, I had no place I could really be me. The only place I could go was my hometown. And I knew that would break me.

I lived with Mum for a while, but it didn't work out. She held loud phone conversations late at night; I went out without saying when I'd be back. Over time, our arguments grew more and more frequent, and I grew to dread being at home. I knew that I couldn't deal with it, and wanted better. One day, I decided enough was enough, and simply walked out.

I didn't know where I was going, but I couldn't stay in my shitty hometown. I'd been offered a job in retail, and I just knew that's where I'd end up staying for the rest of my life if I accepted it. I wanted more than that. I didn't know how, and I knew that just running away with no plan wouldn't solve anything, but I had to go. Anything was better than giving up on life before I'd even started.

My relationship with Jasper wasn't quite dead. After we'd broken up, we'd see other people, then periodically get back together and go through the whole break-up process all over again. Yet, somehow, we kept gravitating back towards each other.

We were broken up when I turned up at his house that evening, but I didn't know where else to go. I just knew that Exeter was over for me now, my hometown wasn't an option ... I had nothing left. I found myself sitting on a bench at the end of his road, sending a text to Kate to explain what was happening. A few minutes later, she emerged from the flat and walked down the road to take a seat next to me.

'Jasper won't be happy you're here. But you can stay tonight. Just tonight. You need to work out what you're doing.'

I texted Mum to tell her I was staying with Jasper for a while, and by some miracle, I managed to stay on his sofa for a week while I sent out job applications. After a few days, I received a call from a call centre in Exeter. They were desperate for people to join their emergency helpline, taking calls for a tumble dryer company who were recalling models that had been catching fire.

Once I secured the job offer, I spent hours trawling the net, looking for a place I could move into fairly quickly. To my intense surprise and relief, I found a place on the outskirts of the city that a girl was desperate to leave. Her desperation didn't ring any alarm bells for me, as I was desperate myself. I arranged a meeting for the next day, signed a contract, and before I knew it, I was set.

Two days later, I was sitting on the stripped mattress in my new home. It felt weird. I had a room of my own again. I had a job.

After a few hours, I felt lonely, and vaguely afraid. Would I get on with the other housemates? What if I froze up and didn't know what to say, or said the wrong thing?

I'd managed to skirt out to the bathroom and back a few times, but on the third occasion, I heard a knock on my door not long after I'd dived back into my room.

Cautiously, I cracked open the door, and was greeted with a woman dressed in PJs and trainers.

'Hey, could you hold the door open while I climb in through the front window? I'll get locked out if it shuts behind me.'

I must have looked at her like she was crazy, because she laughed. 'Oh, don't worry, I live here. I live ... opposite you? You just moved in, right? I'm Tara.'

I shook her hand, still suspicious. She shook her head, smiling.

'I'll show you. I left my key in my room and shut the door like an idiot. Come on.'

I silently followed her out to the front of the house, and held the chair as she climbed up onto it and squeezed through the top of the window. A crash and muffled 'ouch!' later, she yelled that I could bring the chair back in.

She was holding her door open, a key held triumphantly in her hand. 'Told ya.'

I smiled despite myself.

*

A few weeks later, and I was settled into my call centre job. It wasn't the most challenging of environments – in fact, I was bored out of my mind. My colleagues and I were a real eclectic mix though – the tumble dryer company must have been desperate!

Once we'd learnt the script to regurgitate to customers, all that was left to do was wait. There were such long pauses between calls that I was being paid £7 an hour to sit at a desk, wearing a headset and reading a book or magazine. Some people coloured in. Others were doing their GCSE workbooks at the table.

Then I'd go home, hang out with Tara, smoke weed and stand on the trampoline with her, jumping up and down and screeching at the trains that sped past every 30 minutes directly above our heads.

'Fuck off, ya wankers!' we'd screech, giving the carriages the finger, then collapsing onto the trampoline, laughing hysterically.

It was a life ... of sorts.

The last time I'd smoked weed had been with Joel. He'd always managed to have a stash on him. I'd felt a little uncomfortable the first time he offered me some, but he said it was basically like smoking a cigarette, except the buzz felt better. Cautiously, I took a small drag. Then another. Suddenly, I was floating away on a cloud.

Ahh. How could I have not known about this before? This was great. I didn't have a care in the world when I was high. Joel and I would sit giggling at nothing in my room after a few joints, then rush up to the kitchen and make ridiculous snacks to stuff into our faces. Occasionally, Chris and Hayley would raise their eyebrows at us, but for the most part, they said nothing.

Tara smoked a lot of weed. She was on semi-permanent leave from her job due to severe back issues, and she did bongs in her room, or the garden, to distract from the emotional and physical pain she felt.

It wasn't long before I was doing the same. All it took was picking up a cheap £5 bong of my own, and getting some weed off Tara on a regular basis. Then I got to float away on a cloud whenever I wanted. Being high was much better than having flashbacks, feeling panicky, sitting down and thinking about how shit life was, or coping with the nightmares.

I soon realised the house I'd moved into was basically a cross between a doss house and a playground. Everyone in the area had a key to the front door, it would appear. Even the landlord knew it was a free-for-all. Why didn't he change the lock? Who knows? Maybe he didn't care.

This basically meant that anybody and everybody would walk into the house ... or they'd go for the less traditional method.

The trampoline wasn't just used for screeching at passing trains – often, it was used as a landing strip for anyone who wanted to vault over the fence to get into the house. I'd regularly walk out back to see people vaulting into the garden, or the local drug dealer vaulting into one of the back rooms through the window. He wasn't technically allowed in the house – he'd lived here before, and been banned by the landlord because he'd decided he couldn't be fucked to pay the rent for six months.

Then, one night, I met Jim for the first time. He stumbled out back with a glass of wine in his hand and stared up at the stars. Then he clocked that I was sitting directly behind him, stubbing out a cigarette, and frowned.

'Hang on, do you live here?'

'Er, yeah. Do you?'

'Fucking hell, how many people does Rick cram into this godforsaken house. Yeah, I live upstairs. What do you do?'

'I work at the call centre, lived in Exeter on and off for a while – did my BA here last year.'

'Oh no way, I'm actually doing my MA at the uni, in international relations.'

And so the conversation flowed; we talked about everything from philosophy to his favourite spots in Cape Town – he was from South Africa, and as he talked, I could hear the hint of a buried accent, partly forgotten by years spent in the UK. We stood out back together, staring up at the stars.

*

Before too long, I decided I was done with working at the call centre, listening to strangers scream at me down the phone about their tumble dryer that had randomly caught fire. I wanted more from life.

I sent out more job applications, to the university and elsewhere, and before too long, some of my old lecturers realised I was back in town. I got a call one afternoon, offering me a place on the graduate scheme, working in project management. I remember hanging up the phone with a massive smile on my face, walking back into the call centre and asking to meet with the assistant manager.

'Susie, I'm leaving,' I told her.

'You got another job or something?' she said, idly picking her nails.

'Yep. I'm a project officer at the university.'

She looked up in surprise. 'Good on you, girl. To be honest, I'll be straight – I know this job isn't much cop. If you want to leave now, I wouldn't blame you.'

I paused. 'You mean I can leave right this minute?'

Susie shrugged. 'Why not? Some other desperate bugger will want the position you've left open. And I'll give you a reference if you need it.'

And with that, I got up, grabbed my bag and left the building. I was moving on to bigger and better things.

*

Tara, Jim, and I celebrated with wine that night, out in the shed. It wasn't actually a shed, it was a tiny conservatory rammed with mismatched chairs, a big table, and a tiny heater in the corner.

Before too long, Tara made her excuses and left. 'I'll leave you two alone,' she said, winking at me.

I rolled my eyes. Tara were so desperate for the two of us to get it on. 'Look, you could do with a rebound after your ex. What could possibly go wrong?' she asked innocently one evening.

'Er, a lot of things. For example, I'd be sleeping with my housemate. What if that, you know, ends in heartbreak, and I still have to hang around him every single day because he lives down the hall?' I'd said.

Tara shrugged. 'Would be top lol for the rest of us.'

I sighed.

That night, Jim and I ended up in front of our favourite TV show together. We didn't get it on, but from then on, we were pretty close friends.

We had a routine going – each morning, I'd grab my cigarettes and head out back, knocking on Jim's door as I went. Sometimes I'd catch him shirtless or, even better, he'd head out to the kitchen without his top on.

After chain smoking and downing coffee, we'd walk up to the uni together. During lunch, we'd sometimes meet up, get food, and talk. And later, we'd walk home together, cook together, put on our usual TV show, and relax. The routine was almost always the same. We were acting like an obsessed married couple. It was intense. But I was happy.

And then one night, I looked up at Jim and saw him gazing intently at me. I knew that look. It was what I'd been waiting for.

'Go on, then,' I whispered.

And he kissed me.

CHAPTER 12

MOURNING

The days began to blur into one of the few periods of my life I'd call genuinely happy. A few of my old uni friends were still in Exeter, and we reconnected, so I had a job, a place, friends, and a relationship. It was blissful, and I felt like I belonged.

As time went on, I opened up to Jim about what I'd been through, and even though he couldn't imagine going through it himself, he was supportive and I felt accepted for the first time.

But nothing lasts forever, and my happiness soon started fading away.

I was starting to get acid reflux. That was highly unusual, because I'd never had it before. I was also getting incredibly tired and found it difficult to focus on what was going on around me.

Then my period was late.

A week later, I felt sick to my stomach. I knew what was going on. I wondered if it could be Jim's, but we always used a condom.

I couldn't be sure, but a gut feeling told me whose it was...

I thought about the one night I'd spent with Jasper that last time before I left for good. One thing had led to another. We hadn't used protection.

I walked to the nearest pharmacy in a trance, and bought a pregnancy test. The blue line was faint, but it was definitely there. I was pregnant.

There was no way I could have a child. I was 22, working a fairly low-paid job; I wasn't ready for a child. No, I couldn't do it.

The bundle of cells in my body wasn't a sentient being. It wasn't ... alive. It wouldn't feel pain if I got it ... sucked out. I had to do it. It was the kindest thing to do.

But if that was the case, why did it make me feel like a murderer?

*

Four weeks later, I sat in a waiting room. The room was full of girls who I imagined looked just as I felt – tired, withdrawn, grey-faced. We sat in silence, waiting for our name to be called. I'd taken the day off work to get my pregnancy terminated. Then an alarm went off.

We all raised our heads. The women at the reception desk didn't look too concerned. One of them looked up. 'It's just a routine thing, happens every day,' she told us.

Our heads went back down. But within a few minutes, it started getting annoying. This was already the worst day of our lives. Now we had to listen to a bloody siren going off while we waited for the most harrowing part of it.

There was a red button on the wall next to the reception desk that read 'Turn off alarm'. I wondered why the receptionists hadn't done it. Then I realised they were probably so used to the sound, it barely registered anymore. I wondered if I'd get away with just walking over there and hitting the button. I was itching to do it, but I didn't quite have the guts.

Then I saw a girl much younger than me march irritably over to the button. She couldn't have been more than 16, and she looked pissed. She thwacked the button, and the siren stopped. We all looked up in relief and smiled at her. She smiled back and took her seat.

*

There were so many people milling around in the preparation room. I was lying on a hospital bed, trying not to have a panic attack. The doctors all looked confident and friendly; like they'd done this a million times before. But I knew I was about to be put to sleep for the procedure, and I was freaking out. I'd never had an operation like this before. What if the drugs didn't work? What if I woke up halfway through and had to actually see the ... foetus (I cringed) being pulled out of me?

My breathing got quicker, shallower. A doctor noticed and turned to me. 'This will be fine. Women go through this procedure every single day. Just lie back and think of something nice.' Then he turned away again.

Easy for him to say. He wasn't about to get knocked out and have a living thing sucked out of him.

I briefly thought about getting up, walking away from the preparation room, running out of the hospital. Getting into a taxi, going home. Remaining pregnant. Having a baby. Doing the right thing. Giving life to a bunch of cells who deserved it. I'd done this, after all. I had to see it through.

I pictured the baby I'd hold in my arms. Would she have big blue eyes, like mine? Would he have thick tufts of muddy brown hair, like Jasper? Would she be quiet, like I'd been? Or would he be full of energy, a screamer?

My heart warmed as I thought about cradling my child, rocking her to sleep. Watching him sleep. Watching her play. Taking him to school. I could be a mother. I knew I could. I could have a child. A child of my own. To love and care for. Forever. I wouldn't have to run away anymore. I'd have a little person who loved me. Who needed my care. And I could do that. I could be a mum.

'This is going to sting a bit, but you'll soon be feeling sleepy. Let yourself fall asleep, it's totally normal,' the doctor said, pushing a needle into the back of my hand.

I thought about what would happen if I just went back to my room and remained pregnant. I'd have a child, who needed nappies, food, constant attention. I'd have to give up my job. I'd need to claim benefits. I would be on my own, for years, looking after a child. I would want to run away, and I wouldn't be able to. Then I saw myself putting my child to sleep, and pouring pills into my mouth. Social services putting the baby in care. The child growing up to hate their irresponsible, druggie mother who never cared about them.

An oxygen mask was placed over my face, and my eyes fluttered open. Everyone was looking down at various parts of my body, sticking needles into me. I felt a rush of cold fear. I couldn't do this. I couldn't ... do this ...

I woke up in the corner of a large room, curtained off to give me privacy. I hadn't felt this awake in weeks. Then I looked down at my hospital gown, and remembered.

The baby was gone.

I felt wet between my legs, and lifted up the gown. A pool of blood was gathering at my crotch. I remembered the nurse telling me I'd bleed a lot for a few weeks afterwards, and that I'd need to bring sanitary pads to the hospital with me. I got up, and sorted myself out. I could feel the bleeding. It was worse than any period I'd had. It felt like my body was mourning. It had lost something it wanted to grow, to cherish, to love.

I realised I was crying. I was mourning, too.

In the weeks that followed, I slowly told Tara and Jim what had happened. Their support meant the world to me. Sometimes I had nightmares about my ghost child coming back to seek revenge, and it was hard. I would go to Jim's room during those nights, because I couldn't bear to be alone.

When the new year dawned, I decided it was time to start afresh. I felt ready to start a new chapter, but fate decided to hurl another obstacle in my path ...

CHAPTER 13

I CAN'T BREATHE

It all started with a cough.

And mould.

As the winter wore on, more and more black spores appeared on my walls. Everyone told me to simply wipe the spores off the wall, which I did – but they came back every few hours, so by the morning, I'd wake up coughing and hacking up all sorts of disgusting stuff.

Smoking soon became difficult, and lowering my intake of nicotine did not make me a happy bunny. We all have our vices, and mine was sitting out back with either a spliff or a cigarette, watching the stars and listening to music. But even that was taken away from me.

I asked Rick if he could do something about it, and he told me the room had been newly refurbished, and there were no problems with it – damp was a common problem, and I should just crack open a window.

'Crack open a fucking window?' I told Jim one night, as we sat with pizza and a movie on my bed. 'This window is massive and opens out onto the main road. He's telling me to go out to work and leave all my possessions open to getting nicked!'

Everyone in the house knew I had a bad cough by that point. Two French girls we lived with, Adele and Sophie, were all too aware of the issues in my room.

'I felt ill in there when I had it six months ago,' Adele told me out in the shed one night. 'And the girl in there before you argued with Rick over the mould problem, then left pretty quickly.'

I got a feeling Rick just didn't care if I got ill, as long as he got his money.

'He loves getting dollar,' said a housemate on Facebook. 'I heard him the other morning speaking to a construction worker outside the house, saying the mould problem is back in your room.'

So he knew full well there was a mould problem. I was perplexed. How could someone prioritise money over someone's wellbeing?

Doing bongs wasn't just a way for me to escape by that point. It helped with the pain, because every morning, I was waking up with a chest that burnt, and it felt like I was breathing through a straw.

I got into a routine – open my eyes, push down the panic as I couldn't breathe properly, wait for my airways to clear, cough violently.

Then I'd go to the sink and hack up a lung, throw up, and drink some water. The burning pain in my chest weighed me down, but I tried my best to ignore it. Then I'd walk to work.

When I'd first started the job, the walk up several hills had felt relatively easy, and when I went with Jim, our chats made it quicker. But as I got more and more ill, I started deliberately leaving the house before him. Why? I didn't want anyone to see how ill I was. I'd walk up half a slope, stop to throw up in the street, then carry on for a bit. Then repeat, over and over, until I got into work.

I had to spend as much time as I could away from my room, so when I returned home from my little office, I'd sit in the garden, or listen to smooth jazz in Jim's room, then we'd cook and hang out with Tara and her snake. But afterwards, I had to go to my room. I'd tried sharing Jim's bed, but he only had a single and whenever we slept in it together, one of us would suddenly wake up on the floor. So back to my own bed I went … resigning myself to the pain all over again.

It wasn't long, though, before Jim saw just how bad things had become.

One evening, I stumbled out of the shower, coughing and wheezing. My chest had tightened up, and I felt incredibly weak. Jim jumped to his feet when he saw me collapsed on the floor.

'Imi. Imi, are you awake?' I could feel him gently shaking me, but I couldn't get together the energy to respond. He gently picked me up.

'Look, let's get you back to your room. Come on.' He propped me against him, and we half-walked, half-stumbled down the hallway. I kept gasping for air, my eyes rolling back into my head. I couldn't remember ever having felt that helpless.

He got me into bed, and looked down at me, concern clouding his piercing blue eyes. 'Are you going to be okay?'

By this point, I was conscious enough to register embarrassment, and nodded faintly. I tried to speak, and failed. I just gave him a thumbs-up, put the duvet over my head, and waited for sleep to take me.

I could feel him standing over me for a few minutes longer, clearly unsure if he was safe to leave or not. Then he sighed, and I heard the gentle click of my door closing behind him.

As the months went by, my hours went part-time, and I shifted into doing extra part-time work at a clothes shop. The hours were long, the work was tough, and I was exhausted at the end of each day.

I partied, I drank, I did drugs, and I spent a lot of my time blocking out the pain of living through what I would realise, later in life, was mould poisoning. But at the time, nobody knew what it was. My housemates overheard me coughing up a lung in the morning, and presumed I was just smoking too much. My GP, however, had other thoughts.

When my breathing got so bad I could barely walk up the slopes to work, I booked a day off and went to the doctors. By that point, the coughing was near constant, and it got worse whenever I walked. So, the 20-minute walk to the surgery probably wasn't the best idea. When I arrived, I felt awful sitting in the waiting room – and when my name was called, I walked into the doctor's office, strolled to the sink and threw up in it.

'Well, you're clearly not feeling too great,' the doctor remarked as I sat down in the seat opposite him.

After asking me some questions, he said I'd need to go for a scan to rule out the big C. Specifically, lung cancer ... I went home and told Jim. His eyes widened.

'Shit, how are you feeling?'

'I dunno. I mean, if it's cancer, it's cancer, you know? I'm not really scared of death. What's the point? If this is when I'm meant to go, it is what it is.'

Easter rolled around, and Jim told me to take his room for the fortnight he'd be visiting his parents.

'You have to sort that room out. I don't think you can take getting much worse than you already are.'

So I shifted down the hallway, spent a few nights in his broken bed, and woke up one morning with my airways completely clear. Right. That was it. I had to tackle this ...

I walked into my room, armed with bleach, cleaning wipes and sprays, protective masks, and gloves. Opening the window, I pulled the mask over my face and got to work.

I coughed and opened the window wider. I could barely breathe; the amount of mould was so extreme. I pulled the bed frame out from the corner of the room, and almost threw up. Layer upon layer of mould in varying shades of green, black, and brown coated the bottom half of three walls. The wall crumbled away, and a group of spiders scuttled out of one hole and into another. My stomach churned. I had to clean the mould off the wall. I had no choice. This was the only time window I had to fix it.

I covered the floor with tarpaulin and tightened my air mask. I put on a thick pair of gloves, got the cleaners out, extended an arm, and sprayed. The smell was overwhelming. I coughed, and leant forwards. I scrubbed the wall. I kept scrubbing. I coughed, sucked in the little air I could, hung my head out the window to take in fresh oxygen, then scrubbed some more.

Half an hour later, I was down to the bottom layer. My eyes were stinging and streaming. Suddenly, my throat seized up. Not only was I struggling to see, now I couldn't breathe, either. I stumbled to my feet and fell across my room. Air. I needed air. Clean air. Oxygen. Breathing. I needed to breathe again.

Breathe in ...

I fell into the corridor and collapsed on the floor. The house was silent – no one was there to help me. The more I tried to breathe, the more my throat seized up. My head was spinning. I was choking on vomit. I wiped my streaming eyes with the back of my arm, but they wouldn't stop stinging. I couldn't see. I still couldn't breathe.

The next few seconds lasted a lifetime. Everything slowed down. I rolled onto my back, looked up at the ceiling, and breathed in, very slowly. It didn't work. I couldn't get air into my system. I was suffocating on the mould that had been slowly poisoning me for six months. The spores had been disturbed by my scrubbing, and now ... I didn't know if I was going to make it.

I knew I wasn't afraid of death. And as I lay on the floor, unable to breathe, my face and throat swollen, I came to terms with the fact that maybe I wouldn't take in another clear breath. Maybe I'd die there and then. But if I survived ... I was going to do what I wanted to do with my life.

In that moment, I realised life was for living to the full, and I knew that if I got out of this, I was going to follow my dreams. I was going to write for a living. I would become a journalist. I would find a way to make it happen.

I breathed in, and it was enough. It hurt – God, it hurt so much – but I got enough air into my system. I breathed in again, ignored the pain, and sat up. I wiped my eyes, and breathed in. I was going to make it. I was okay. Goddammit, I was okay. This wasn't going to beat me. I was going to finish cleaning that mould.

Then I blacked out.

*

The paramedic took my temperature. Tara stood behind him, looking worried. I realised she must have discovered me and called for help.

I was running a fever. 'Let's get you out of this room. Now. It's a health and safety hazard.' I couldn't speak. I just nodded.

'Aren't you going to take her to hospital?' Tara demanded.

The paramedic looked hesitant. 'We could, but it's incredibly busy there tonight. She'd just be sitting in a waiting room for several hours. Honestly, it'd be better for you if you went somewhere dry and warm right now, and got some sleep. You can call emergency again in the morning if your symptoms worsen.'

Tara nodded reluctantly, then helped me to Jim's room. I shut my eyes and let sleep take me.

The next morning, I woke up and tried to breathe. It was like inhaling through a straw that had been sealed shut. I forced in as much air as I could, coughed, spluttered, and threw up all over the bed. Then I gasped for air. My eyes were still stinging. I could feel my swollen throat. I tried to speak. Nothing but a hoarse squeak came out. I lay back on the bed and cried. Getting better was going to take a long time. I couldn't move. I couldn't speak. I knew the only option right now was to rest, keep drinking fluids, and pray I'd make it.

For 10 days I sat in Jim's room, unable to breathe, see properly, speak, or think coherent thoughts. I texted Tara each morning and evening to let her know I was okay. I was too embarrassed to let her see me, and couldn't face sitting in a hospital. If I was going to get better, it was going to be on my own.

I listened to films, sipped on hot liquids, and slept a lot. Sometimes I'd wake up to a coughing fit, then throw up in the sink. Every day, it got a little easier to breathe.

On the 10th day, I woke up and breathed in. I inhaled, and the air came rushing in. Tears filled my eyes. I was going to be okay.

Since that day, I haven't feared death. I looked it in the face when I was lying on the ground, struggling to breathe. Then I walked away, ready to start again.

CHAPTER 14

TIME TO RUN AWAY

Now that I'd been given a second chance, I wasn't going to hold back. I spent my evenings applying like crazy to jobs in London, speaking with recruiters, and tweaking my CV so it looked perfect.

A few weeks later, I got an email from the managing editor at a huge media company. She was looking for an intern to work at their Shoreditch office for three months. The pay wasn't great, but it would get my foot in the door. It was my big chance, so I grabbed it.

I passed the written test, got the bus to London and attended a two-hour interview. Everything went well, and I felt like maybe life was finally going my way.

On my way home, I got a phone call from the editor, and she offered me the job. I was ecstatic. All my hard work at university had paid off. Getting through the mould poisoning had been worth it. I had a path. I knew what I was going to do with my life.

That afternoon, I celebrated with Jim and Tara in the shed, doing bongs and drinking wine.

But just as I was starting to let the happiness seep through me, my phone rang again. It was the editor.

'Hi, Imogen? Hey, hope you're doing well. I just wanted to tell you something, and this isn't easy for me to say. We've just had a big meeting with the MD, and he wants to take the company in a totally different direction. We really like you, and this is no reflection on you, but he wants to pull the internship ...'

My dreams shattered.

A cold, sick feeling spread through my entire body. The happiness that had been overflowing just minutes before drained out of me.

Hanging up the phone, I got up and left the shed, ignoring Tara and Jim's confused protests. I got into bed, pulled the covers over me, and didn't emerge again for three days.

*

There was a shuffling sound coming from underneath my bedroom door. My eyes snapped open in a surge of fear. Was somebody trying to get in?

A brown envelope suddenly appeared. Someone had shoved a letter under my door. I grabbed it and took it back to bed. I was glad I was sitting down when I opened it. The sickness I'd felt just days earlier was back. The letter was from my landlord; he'd found out I'd cleaned the mould from the wall, and was adamant that I'd broken the tenancy agreement by carrying out my own repairs. He was evicting me. I had just over a month to get out.

The Mad Traveller sat up and stretched. Her Cupboard was covered in cobwebs, and the door creaked as it opened. She was stiff, groggy, but awake.

Was it time to run away again?

I felt nothing but cold fear. I had to run away. I wasn't escaping, I was being forced away and there was nothing I could do about it. School was over. Uni was over. My jobs were ending. There was nothing for me in my hometown, or my dad's place. Jasper had disappeared a long time ago. Jim would be moving away soon, once his MBA was over. Life was rolling on, and I was being pushed out.

I could feel myself free falling, like the night I'd fallen from the stranger's car. But this time, there was no bus ready to pick me up and take me home. I had nowhere to go. There was nowhere I belonged.

I couldn't drift away anymore. I couldn't just ... escape. I had to do it right. But how? How was I going to forge the future I wanted?

I opened my laptop and got to work.

*

'So you're really leaving soon, then,' Jim said, taking a drag on his cigarette.

We were in the garden. I waited to speak as a train rumbled above our heads.

'Yeah, I guess I am,' I replied. I hadn't really thought about it. Giving it too much attention made it scary, and I couldn't afford to chicken out.

I'd applied for a bank loan, and breathed a sigh of relief when £5,000 had appeared in my account. I didn't know how I'd pay it back, but I couldn't worry about that right now. I'd pay it back, one day. When I was settled.

Now that I had money, I could look for somewhere to live, and start applying for jobs again. Any job, in London. No other city really made sense to move to. If I wanted to work in the media, I had to place myself in the capital.

I thought about the days in school I'd spent daydreaming about living in the capital, having a glamorous life. At the time, the big city had felt like a glitzy dream world. Now, it just felt terrifying. But if I was going to have a future, I had to get a job in London. And because nothing was going my way, I was going to have to force it. It was now or never.

I tried to think about the times I'd felt unable to cope when I was younger. I'd wanted to just run away. I visualised what I'd dreamt of achieving, once I was away from all the stuff that was making my head hurt. I had always dreamt of London. I was good at journalism. I could make those two things work. If I ran away properly, I could escape a bad situation and make it good. I didn't have to lose myself. I could find myself.

*

Finding a spare room in London is easy enough if you have the right amount of money to throw at a landlord. I scheduled in several house viewings over a single day, then took an early coach across the country and braced myself for a hectic day.

Riding the Underground by myself was scary. I was used to small, slow trains on the south coast, and buses that appeared once every hour – if you were lucky – in my rural hometown. But the sound of underground trains was terrifying. I stood on the platform and felt my stomach churn as the rumbling sound of the approaching train got closer and closer. How did people just wait, so calmly, without having panic attacks?

By some miracle, I made it to my viewings, and one of the rooms looked good enough that I could picture myself in it. I told the landlord I was interested, sat myself down in a coffee shop and connected to the dodgy Wi-Fi so I could wire over a deposit. I prayed that I wasn't being screwed over. In a week, I'd be taking a huge suitcase across the city, setting myself up in a tiny room in East London, and applying like crazy for jobs until something worked out.

What else could I do?

*

The last person I said goodbye to was Jim. It was all a bit last minute, in the end.

On the day I was planning to leave, I got a heads-up from Tara that Rick was heading over to move a new tenant in. The last thing I wanted to do was be there while he was around. What if he came in and saw that I was clearly moving out without telling him?

I was only going to hand in my notice when I was sure I could definitely get into my new room in London – and I knew I wasn't going to be screwed over by my new landlord. There was still a lot of stuff I had to shift across the country, and I couldn't afford to spend a wad of cash on removals companies, so I was going to travel by coach between Exeter and London with a loaded suitcase once a week until the room was empty.

Having a showdown with Rick, then, wasn't the best idea. I hastily booked a taxi and asked Jim if he'd help me with my bags. He took my suitcase and walked out with me to where the taxi was waiting.

Our time had run out, and I had to say goodbye to the last person who'd made my final stint in Exeter worthwhile. It was the end of an era – the two of us dealing with living in a shit-heap under a landlord who ignored us.

'You're doing the right thing,' he told me, as I got into the taxi.

'I know. I'll be okay.'

'You always are.'

Three weeks later

Raul was ... an enthusiastic kind of guy. He'd rung me up the previous week saying he had an amazing opportunity for me. He'd read over my CV, and knew I was the perfect candidate for the role. He couldn't tell me anymore though; I just had to meet him in Soho.

And so I'd rushed to meet him, believing that this recruiter could solve all my problems and offer me a job in the City. After all, I'd seen other people from uni get into work just a few months after graduating. It had been a year since I'd completed my degree, and I'd done so much outside of my work to gain experience in journalism. Surely I was in with a chance?

When I sat down, Raul looked me up and down. 'Don't leave your drink on the table.'

I put it in my pocket, frowning.

'Alright, so run me through your CV.'

I repeated the information that he was looking at. Now it was his turn to frown.

'Don't just regurgitate what's on the page to an employer, alright. Or at least, if you do, add something else in to liven it up a bit.'

I was confused. Why was I being criticised the moment I walked through the door?

'Okay, so if I do pass you on to my client ...' (Hang on, he'd said I was the perfect candidate) ... 'You'll need to look the part. Do you own a suit?'

'What?'

'You'll need to take the nose piercing out. And if you can hide the eyebrow one, that'd be good.'

I was completely taken aback. First my experience wasn't good enough, and now I didn't look right, either?

My piercings and hair colour didn't stop me from doing my job, so what did it matter?

Apparently it did matter.

'It's very professional. Big, big clients. Global clients. You have to look corporate.'

This was news to me. I'd spent the last six months walking into the offices at my university to work in whatever I liked, and it had just been accepted. Now I had to dress up?

'Alright, I reckon I'll pass you on to them. If you sort your hair and piercings out, you'll be fine, you obviously know your stuff.'

I wandered back into Soho in a daze. What was I meant to do? Did I really have to change how I looked to fit in?

I looked at all the suits rushing past and sighed.

When I got back to my little room in East London, I headed to the bathroom and took a good, long look at myself in the mirror.

Was I willing to let go of my appearance for a chance at having a future?

I took my nose ring out.

*

One of my friends from uni got in touch once she heard I was in London. She was working as a producer on a daytime TV show, and suggested I come along to be a part of the audience. 'It'll give you a distraction from job applications,' she said with a smile.

So one morning, I took the Tube over to the studio. Everyone I spoke to was lots of fun, and I was surprised to find myself feeling totally comfortable. I got on particularly well with a man called Eli, who was quirky, interesting, and funny, and figured I could probably come back the next day ...

Another friend dropped me a message a few hours later. 'Are you near East London?' she wanted to know.

'Yes ... it's where I live.'

'This woman from Channel 4 is looking for people to be in the audience of her political show tonight.'

'Yeah, why not?'

This was nuts! Two TV shows in one day? It was such a crazy coincidence. But then, life had been getting more and more crazy ...

Ten minutes later, I got a call from ITN, then my email confirmation was sent through. Before I knew it, I was on the Tube again.

Once the show was over, I noticed model and TV personality Katie Price standing with her entourage backstage. Acting on impulse, I asked her for a photo, then headed back to the Tube, buzzing with adrenaline. TV and celebrities – London was a whole world away from sleepy little Exeter.

Even at one o'clock in the morning, this part of the city, flanked by the HSBC and Barclays skyscrapers, was vibrant, full of life. I jogged through the streets to the Underground as lightning struck; thunder rumbled and rain began to pour. Everyone was scrambling for cover as the storm chased people under cover.

I got into Greenwich and waited for my train. The rain was still pouring like there was no tomorrow. I wondered vaguely if this was an omen of what was to come, then told myself I'd had too much to drink, put my earphones in, and forgot about it.

*

Life started ticking over in a strange new way. I spent my mornings in the TV studio, as there was always plenty of room to be in the audience. I hung out with Eli and my other new friends, then spent my afternoons in job interviews. I was worried about money, so I logged an application for Universal Credit, the new benefits allowance that was being rolled out for the first time in parts of London. I was in a trial area, and I hoped the new monthly allowance, which included housing, wouldn't impact on my tenancy – I was trying my best to make out like I was employed, from fear of being evicted for having no income, and I deliberately stayed out of the house most of each day.

I hadn't had any success with job interviews, but I figured it was just a numbers game. And besides, maybe going on Universal Credit would be a good thing – they would help me find a job, even if I was stuck cleaning toilets for a while. Then at least I'd have regular money coming in while I worked out my next move.

I hadn't heard much from my new landlord, but at the start of August, he knocked on my door.

'The downstairs tenants are saying the water from the bathroom leaks through their ceiling when you shower. Could you keep an eye on that, please?'

That was news to me. I hadn't been aware there was any problem. Then the landlord paused, and looked hesitant.

'Also ... I wanted to discuss something, but I can see you're in a rush, so maybe another time.' I had my jacket on as I was planning to head up north and see Eli for the afternoon.

'No, it's fine, what is it?'

'I've had an offer from some people who really need a new place to stay. They're good friends of mine, and they need to move by next month. I was wondering if you'd be able to pack up your stuff and leave by September. I just don't think it's going to work. You know, the water leaking through and stuff, innit.'

My brain started pumping out questions to consider. Could I go to the council and get him done for illegal eviction? Probably, but the process would take weeks and create even more stress for me when I already had enough going on. Could I argue? Yes, but I didn't want to get into a fight with a man six inches taller than me. Should I just move again? That seemed like it would be the easiest option. I was fairly sure he'd try to pin disrepair charges on me for "having water leak through the ceiling" if I tried to contest it, anyway. After the Exeter landlord, I didn't trust anyone who rented out rooms to people for extortionate prices.

Outwardly, I was silent. Emotionally, I didn't feel anything. I found that interesting, and idly contemplated why that may be. Then I realised I was so accustomed to pain, now, that I had none left to feel.

'I have nowhere to go. I'd have to ask my friend if I can sleep at his place.'

'Yeah, when would that be?' he asked eagerly.

'I don't know, he's gone away for a month,' I said, trying to buy myself some time. 'I can see if I can leave mid-September, if you want.'

'Yeah, let me know, alright.' The conversation was clearly over.

I put my headphones on and turned the volume up.

*

The fear started to set in once he'd left. I wondered how I was supposed to get it together and head out to meet Eli. I felt like I'd finally been getting back on my feet, only to be knocked down once again.

The neighbours were having a party. I couldn't hear myself think. I got dressed and left the house.

Half an hour later, I stepped off the Tube. I was still struggling, so I messaged Eli to say I needed to sit in the park for a while before I headed over.

When I eventually made it to his place, he answered the door with a massive smile on his face. He ushered me inside, and I talked in more depth about what had happened.

'Well, here's a suggestion for you. Why don't you come and live with me? I know we barely know each other, but we'd be banding against these bastard landlords who use people.

You'll only need to pay me £40 a week, so you can save money, I'll save money; we're all winners.' He beamed at me, and much as I knew I was playing with fire, I accepted.

It was a simple choice: go back home to nothing, live on the streets, or live with Eli. I so desperately wanted to make a future for myself that I was willing to take a huge risk. I knew I was putting myself in danger, but my life had already been so full of dangerous situations, I had a pretty loose grip on what danger really meant by that point. It felt as if the future I wanted was so close at hand. If I went home, I had no future. If I didn't make it, I had no future. The only option that could give me a future was living with Eli.

Diary – 3rd August 2016

I'm shifting my stuff over to Eli's place in a few days. I won't be giving my landlord his final month of rent – he can get fucked. He's illegally evicting me, so why should I pay him to do that? I'm just going to leg it out of here with my suitcase during the day, when no one else is in the house to notice I've scarpered.

I never thought, when I moved here, that I'd be arranging to share a bedsit with a man I barely know, just so I can keep a roof over my head while I find my feet here.

It worries me, still, of course. Eli could easily stop messaging me, stop turning up to the TV studio, and I'd be facing looking at hostels in a few weeks. But we've connected, over the last few weeks – I don't think he'd do that to me. I find it hard to trust people, after what I've been through, but for some reason, I still have the capacity to do so. And I trust Eli.

CHAPTER 15

THIS IS ROCK BOTTOM

Hidden away in the hustle and bustle of London is the Islington canal. When you go down the stairs and walk next to the water, all the noise disappears, and you can pretend you're in the middle of nowhere. It's one of my favourite places to go and de-stress.

Since I'd moved to London, I'd been looking for a happy place. I'd had several in Exeter, but now I was hundreds of miles away. I missed the sleepy rhythm of Exeter life, the green fields, the early morning or late evening walks along the river Exe. When Eli had introduced me to the canals, life felt a little easier because I had a place I could go and just ... be.

A few days after learning I'd need to leave my rental, I found myself on the Northern line, heading up to the canals. It was early Saturday morning, so the only other people on the Tube were sleepy commuters on the weekend shift and droopy party-goers from the night before, heading home in their too-tight outfits and sparkly make-up.

Once I was walking along the canal, I breathed an internal sigh of relief. I was meeting Eli in a few hours, so I figured I'd hang out there before going to see him. I took a seat on one of the benches arranged in a semi-circle under a canopy of trees, plugged in my earphones and zoned out, looking at the water and focusing on the beat of the music.

Half an hour later, I registered a man sitting a few benches down from me. He'd appeared so silently, I wondered how long he'd been there without me realising. He was dressed in a long black coat, stained trousers and dirty trainers. My stomach did a funny flip. He didn't exactly look friendly.

A few minutes later, I glanced at him out of the corner of my eye and realised he was looking directly at me. A cold shiver ran down my neck, to the bottom of my spine. What was he doing? Was he planning something? If I left, would he follow me? Could I out-run him? I knew the canals like the back of my hand, so I started thinking of ways I could out-wit him by taking the shortcuts not many people knew about.

The man had started looking at me, then down at his crotch, over and over again. I felt sick. What if he was going to try to force something sexual on me? A memory flashed up in my mind.

I was with him. He wanted me to wrap my lips around his penis. I'd never heard of blowjobs before, and thought the concept was disgusting. But he wanted it, and so I was forced to obey.

Was it about to happen again? I looked back at him, and my heart dropped to my stomach.

He was holding his erect penis in his hand and masturbating, while staring at me.

Before I could process anything further, my body went on auto pilot. I stood up and walked away, cutting through the trees. I heard a rustle behind me, and sped up, not daring to look and see if it was him.

Once I was through the uneven path along the trees, I put my phone in my pocket and started running. There were some back streets I could dart through to get to one of Eli's friends' houses, and once I was there, I'd be safe.

I felt self-conscious about running so quickly, so tried to wipe the look of panic off my face and make out like I was just going for a morning run. I didn't know why that mattered. Surely if someone thought I was in trouble, they'd help, and that was a good thing, but my mind was throwing up random things to focus on, as silly as they might be.

I arrived at Leslie's place, and sat on the porch outside. There was no sign of the man. I waited a few minutes further, then let myself relax. He was gone.

I called Eli, and told him what had happened. He said he'd be over as soon as he could.

I'd been introduced to Leslie a month or so after meeting Eli. One afternoon, I'd had no job interviews to go to, and so he'd suggested we head over to Leslie's place. When we walked in, I realised that she was still in bed, and felt awkward. 'No, it's okay, she's bed-bound. Cancer,' he told me, opening her bedroom door.

The room smelt faintly of sick, and it was clear she was smoking a lot of marijuana. She lay in bed, watching TV, extreme pain written all over her face. I took a deep breath. I hadn't been expecting this, and I didn't know how to behave.

'Hey, Leslie!' Eli beamed, sitting down next to her and getting out some rolling papers. 'I've brought over your latest supply,' he said, pulling out a bud of weed and winking at her.

'Thanks, love ... who's this?' Leslie said faintly, craning her neck to look up at me. I gave a stupid wave as I stood in the doorway, not knowing how to proceed.

'This is my friend Imi. She's come with me to keep you company,' Eli said, smiling at me and gesturing to a chair for me to sit down.

'Ah, that's nice ... make yourself at home, love. Do you want a drink? There's plenty in the kitchen, and there's snacks too, help yourself. Any friend of Eli's is a friend of mine. I'd get up myself, but ...' She looked down at her body, wrapped up in blankets, and chuckled. Her laugh turned into a wheeze, and Eli jumped up to pour her some water from the jug on the windowsill.

'Thank you,' I squeaked, retreating to the kitchen. I hadn't wanted to stay in the bedroom for much longer. I didn't know how to behave, what to say. I'd thought we were just going to a friend's place to watch TV. Well, I guess we were, but ...

Eli joined me next to the fridge. 'Why didn't you tell me?' I said.

'Tell you what? Oh, the cancer. Sorry, sometimes I forget that it's a lot for people to take in.'

'Is it ... terminal? Is she bed-bound?' I asked.

'Yeah. We don't know how long she has left. She has a carer who comes round every day.' Eli checked his watch. 'Yeah, Jen will be here in about 20 minutes, and she helps Leslie go to the toilet, shower, all that stuff.'

'I really shouldn't be here,' I said. I felt so painfully awkward.

'What? No! It's fine. Leslie likes company. She hates being on her own. She's happy you're here. Why don't you come and sit down in the other room? I'm just rolling her some joints ... helps her with the pain, you see.'

I hesitantly walked back into the bedroom with him and took a seat in the rocking chair in the corner. *Judge Judy* was playing on the TV, so I tuned in to that. 'Oh, I've seen this one,' I found myself saying. The conversation started to flow.

I started going to Leslie's place a few times a week with Eli, keeping her company as she watched TV and bringing her snacks from the shop down the road. She told me about how she'd been married, once, but he'd left her. She'd spent a lot of time partying – much too hard – and then found out about the cancer. She had no family left, so Eli was like a son to her. 'I just want the best for him,' she said, smiling down at him.

I wondered how she managed to talk about everything in such a matter-of-fact way. She was only in her late forties, and already in the twilight of her life. A lot had happened to her, but she wasn't letting it get her down. She watched her favourite TV shows, laughed and joked with Eli, and ate her favourite snacks. She seemed to have accepted that it was nearly time for her to go, and she was okay with that.

I thought about my own situation. Things weren't great for me, but I had a whole life ahead of me. This would probably be the hardest part, but if I could smile, find the silver lining where I could, and just get through it, then it would be okay. If Leslie could do it, then I sure as hell could.

Six weeks later

Diary – 17th September 2016

I woke up in a room I didn't recognise about an hour ago. Then I remembered I'm on the fourth floor of a hotel in Kensington.

I can't handle living with Eli anymore. Everything is different now. I don't recognise him. I don't recognise myself anymore.

Whenever I get changed, he looks at me like I'm a delicious snack. It makes me feel so, so uncomfortable. It makes me feel objectified. He just sees me as this sexual plaything for him to look at and enjoy. And every time he crawls over to my mattress and starts tugging at my clothes, stroking me, putting his arms all over me, there's nothing I can do. Can he not see that sometimes I don't want that? Whenever I push his wandering hands away, he starts kissing my neck. 'You wouldn't be so cruel,' he simpers. Then his hands wander again, and I give up.

Every time he stacks up condoms on the cabinet I'm filled with this sense of dread. Every time he comes through the door it's only a matter of time until we're having sex. I don't want to, anymore. I used to, but not since he stopped listening to me – and it's not just in digital messages ... it's when I talk and he rolls his eyes if it doesn't interest him, and turns up his music or videos. I feel like I don't have a voice. Then I take my top off to get changed for bed and he's sitting there gazing at me. Eyes fixated. And I feel sick to my stomach.

I'm being used. He doesn't care what I have to say, but he finds me sexually attractive, so he's got a woman staying in his room who he can climb onto whenever he likes. And there's nothing I can do about it, because I have nowhere to go.

It had been six weeks since I'd moved in with Eli. Every day was the same. Wake up. Pretend to be asleep. Wait for Eli to leave.

Apply for jobs. Check my bank balance, on the off chance it had money in it. Go to McDonald's, wait for families to leave leftover food. Take it.

Ignore the hunger. Wait for Eli to come home. Get raped. Lie on the mattress, reading a book, waiting for the day it finally ends.

It was worse than it had been with him. Nothing had been worse than this. The only thing I had, that remained my own, was my mind. My money, my home, my body, my career, my food ... I wasn't in control of any of it. But I could keep going, every day, until one of the job interviews I attended worked out, and I could earn enough money to leave ...

One night, we had a flaming row. I was sick of him eating in front of me and not offering me anything. I was starving. He told me I should be grateful I had somewhere to live. I'd had enough. I got up and put my phone into my bag. I started putting my shoes on.

'You off, then?'

I didn't respond, and headed to the door.

'Think long and hard. I've done nothing wrong.'

I went to sit in the park over the road. I didn't know what to do.

Everyone seemed to think I was complaining, and apparently, I didn't have that right. When I'd been to the jobcentre earlier, my work coach had signalled for me to come over.

'So how are things after your complaining last week?'

'You mean when I called the service centre because my benefits got cut?'

'Yes ... let's book you in for another "How To Find A Job" seminar.'

In their eyes, if my money got cut, pushing me below the poverty line, and I had an issue with that, it meant I was complaining. In Eli's eyes, if I had an issue with anything about our living situation, I was causing a fight. In their worlds, I should starve, and get ignored, and abused. They'd be cool with that, because they wouldn't have to deal with the consequences of their actions.

Life had never been as bad. I thought about the times I'd wandered to the field, to the bridge, to the streets of London. My life as a lonely teenager. They were all times I'd felt that life had been too much to cope with and I had to escape. But now it felt like I was running out of places to escape to.

I'd been to uni; I'd done everything I was *supposed* to do. I just wanted a job and somewhere to live. But I had run out of options. What was left? Living on the streets?

The Mad Traveller was underwater. Her Cupboard was flooded and she had drowned.

I felt the same burning sensation in my nose that I'd felt that time I'd slipped underwater during a swimming lesson. The same sense of extreme fear; cold panic washing through my stomach and spreading out to the rest of my body. My face hurt; it was filling with water. I couldn't escape. I tried, but I kept sinking. There was no way out.

I was done. I was so done. I felt so alone. I hadn't spoken to any uni friends since before I'd moved to London. They were so busy with their new lives, there was no time to talk anymore. I hadn't spoken to Mum since I'd left her house after graduating. I hadn't spoken to Dad in weeks, and there was no way I could tell him what was really going on. He had started having heart problems, and I wasn't going to be responsible for him having a heart attack. No. I was on my own.

Unless ...

I browsed through the Messenger contacts on my phone. I could talk to Jake. He lived in London, and we talked occasionally. We'd worked on the student paper at uni. I knew he was hating his job at a national, and considering a move to Europe. I didn't know what else to do, so I stopped thinking about it, and just started typing.

A few minutes later, I had a reply.

Jesus, that's awful. Have you talked to anybody about it?

I rang the Samaritans last night because I was so upset and she said, 'The thing that gets me the most is this isn't your fault.' But she didn't know how to solve it. Nobody does. So I hung up.

None of it is your fault, but yeah it is really hard to solve. Have you tried ringing a women's refuge? You can do something to move on tonight if you make yourself do it.

Talking to Jake made me realise I could take charge. I didn't have to let that situation become my life. I could change it.

There weren't any refuge paces available that night, so I was told to ring back the next day.

I messaged my dad, and told him my benefits hadn't come through, and I was low on food. He sent me some money – enough to book a last-minute hotel for the night. That gave me some breathing space. I knew Eli was going to be out the next day, so after he'd gone, I could go and collect my things.

When I got to the hotel I took a long shower. The water in the bedsit was on a timer – whenever I took a shower, I had to put 20-pence pieces into a box, which turned the water on. Then I'd jump in as quickly as possible and get washed before it switched off again. If the water was too hot or too cold, tough luck – spending time adjusting the temperature just wasted the time you'd paid for. So taking a shower without time restrictions – or a group of spiders for company above my head – was bliss.

I had an entire room to myself. I could lock the door, and nobody could come in. It was safe and quiet. I had space to move around in ... and a bed. The clean and comfortable mattress felt so luxurious after sleeping on Eli's thin mattress for so many weeks.

My body was aching so much. My legs were in agonising pain. I was so tired I could barely see straight. Next thing I knew, it was morning.

Time to go back and fight my way out. It was time. I had to stay strong.

CHAPTER 16

FREEDOM

Diary – 1st October 2016

It's been four days. Every day, I've wanted to write about what happened, but each time I've thought about trying, I've not had the right words in my head.

Usually I know what I want to say – the words always come. This time, though, they haven't.

I still don't have the words now, but I feel that I need to force them out. So here goes nothing.

Biscuit wrappers were scattered across the floor of Eli's bedsit. His duvet had been left in a messy heap at the foot of his mattress. The room stank of unwashed clothes, unwashed man, and cannabis.

I climbed onto the kitchen counter and pushed the window open. I took a good look at Eli's mattress for the first time. I'd never realised how filthy it was before. He was sleeping in a filthy, dirty pit. And I'd been forced to do the same for the last two months.

No more. Today marked my last day of living like that. I thought of the hotel room and what it felt like to have a proper bed. My own room. Access to cleaning facilities. Privacy.

It was time to start making calls. I'd find a refuge. I'd leave. For good.

An hour later, and I'd made little progress. Two places said they would call me back, the other three had said there was no room. I scrolled down the list of refuges I'd found on the web. It was ten o'clock. There wasn't much time left.

My phone rang.

'Hi, I'm calling you back from Women's Aid. I've checked with the manager, and we have a room for you.'

She ran through a risk assessment with me. Some of the questions were difficult to answer, and she apologised, but I got through it.

'You'd definitely be eligible to come, and we'd certainly welcome you. When can you get here?'

'I mean, I'm going to be packing a bag once the call is over.'

'In that case, if you could get to the train station, I'll text you with further instructions.'

The call ended. I sat in silence. It was happening. It was really happening.

My phone buzzed with the text.

Hi Imogen, head to the station, see you soon, text me when you are close and I will arrange for someone to come and collect you. Kerry.

I sprang off the mattress and started pulling my belongings out of the cupboard under the sink. I knew I'd have to leave some things behind, but that was okay. The priority was getting out before Eli got back.

My heart was racing. I checked my phone. There was still a bit of time. I started throwing things into my suitcase while I cleaned my teeth, put a bra on, dug out my shoes. Somehow, I was ready in three minutes.

I slowly opened the door. I could hear the guy next door blasting reggae music. The floorboards creaked. He was heading into the corridor. I let the door slide shut, and waited for him to use the bathroom. There was no point in arousing suspicion by having him see me walk out with a suitcase.

I opened the door again. The guy had shut his own. I was safe to leave.

I took one last look at the room, then stepped into the corridor. A gust of wind slammed the door shut, locking it automatically.

If that isn't a sign I was done with the place, I don't know what is!

I wheeled my suitcase to the station. There was a 20-minute wait for my train, and I had to change after half an hour to switch lines, heading east. I prayed I had enough on my Oyster travel card to cover the trip – I couldn't afford to top up.

I was on edge. I knew there was no reason for Eli to be back at this time, but I wouldn't be safe until I was on the train. I watched the boards, wishing time would go by faster. Eventually, the train pulled in, and I dragged my suitcase onboard. I remembered the last time I'd dragged a suitcase onto a train, six years ago and I'd watched from my window as I headed towards Exeter to start a new chapter of my life.

I was starting another new chapter, only this time, I had no idea where I was going.

I'd worked out that my Oyster wouldn't cover the train cost, and I couldn't face being accosted by the security guard waiting at the exit, so I made a snap decision. When he wasn't looking, I quickly dodged the barrier on my way out.

Wheeling my suitcase over the bridge, I felt nervous. What if the whole thing was a wind-up? What if there was no car waiting? I pushed those thoughts to the back of my mind. *No point in entertaining them. Deal with what's in front of you.*

As I walked to the ticket office, a blue Vauxhall drove past and pulled in just ahead of me. A woman got out, and said simply, 'Imogen?'

Kerry introduced herself and helped me load the car with my belongings. Then we headed off.

I was silent. I didn't know what to say. We turned into a quiet, residential road.

'That'll be your house, there – just a normal house. Our office is disguised as another house, just around the corner here.' She turned right, and pulled into the driveway.

It was silent for a moment.

Kerry put her hand on my leg. 'Are you alright? I know it's a lot to take in.'

I hadn't realised I'd been shaking.

'Come on. Let's get you inside.'

Diary – 22nd October 2016

It's been nearly a month since I left him. Really doesn't feel like that long.

I keep checking his Facebook page. I don't know why. It makes me feel properly creepy. I guess I want to know if he's registered the fact I've gone. Not that he'd talk about it on Facebook, but ... oh, I don't know. I can't quite let go yet.

I clicked onto his page this morning. There was a photo of him at a gig. A woman was standing next to him. 'So happy with my beautiful girlfriend who took me out to see my favourite artist!' the caption read.

Life's going on as normal for him, then. He doesn't give a flying fuck that I'm gone. In fact, he's going out with his new girlfriend to gigs. It's as if I never existed. No remorse. No worry for me. Nothing.

Whatever. I don't care. I've got more important things to think about.

Refuge was a safe haven. The women there wanted me to relax, to know that this was my time to heal. I spent a lot of time in my room, watching Netflix, or going for walks into the quiet town centre and wandering around the shops.

I struggled to interact with the other women. I didn't know who to trust. I wasn't sure if they were just going to be the next people to hurt me, or not. I smoked in the garden, with earphones in, so they knew not to disturb me. I knew I was coming across as anti-social, maybe even a bit rude, but I just didn't feel like talking. I wanted to be by myself. Being alone was the only way I felt truly safe.

I'd registered with a new jobcentre, closer to where I lived. There was less pressure on me to find a job, as they were aware of my living situation. For once, I'd been allocated a work coach who was sympathetic. 'I get the sense that you don't have a job right now through no fault of your own,' she told me during our first appointment, while she scanned through my CV. 'I get the impression it's ... circumstantial. Well, we can start afresh now.' She looked up and smiled at me. Hesitantly, I smiled back.

I wasn't able to switch to Jobseekers' Allowance from the Universal Credit I'd been on before – different places, different rules – so I got a living allowance, but no rent. But at least now I was in refuge, I knew I wouldn't be evicted for not paying – they knew it wasn't my fault.

A month after I entered refuge, I was sitting on my bed, filling out job applications. An email pinged into my inbox. It was from Metro.co.uk.

Your CV showed that we would be interested in talking to you about a role we're recruiting for. Would you be interested in having a chat about it?

CHAPTER 17

SEARCH/SEO REPORTER

Are you looking for your gateway into a national publication and / or fascinated by analytics, search metrics and experimenting with new forms of content?

We're looking for a reporter to join our compact search team, to write content that people are searching for and, even better, content our audience will search for in the near future.

Reporters will be expected to work quickly, understand how long a story needs to take to make it what it should be and be able to spot a story that Metro.co.uk should be covering.

If you're interested, let me know and I'll set up a call.

Gabe

I felt something dripping onto my thigh, and realised I was spilling my tea everywhere, I was so engrossed in the email. This was it. *This* was why I'd spent so long going through hell in London. This was the chance I'd been holding on for.

A few hours later, we were on the phone, and as the job was explained to me, I smiled more and more. This would be perfect – if I could get it. How could I stand out from the other candidates, especially considering I had no journalism qualifications? I hadn't been able to afford to take on a diploma or a master's in journalism, so I just had to use what I already had, and hope for the best.

A few days later, I was browsing social media when rapper Azealia Banks popped up on my newsfeed with an update:

To recap my night, I went to a party at Russell Crowe's suite, at which he called me a nigger, choked me, threw me out and spat at me.

Wait, what? I quickly scoured the web to see if anyone was covering the story, then screenshotted the posts in case they got deleted. This could be a story ...

But it was seven o'clock on a Sunday night. Should I take the risk? My gut told me that it would be the kind of thing that would make my application stand out.

I wrote up what I already knew, and messaged Gabe on Twitter.

Ten minutes later, I got a reply.

Email Sarah – this is her address. She's a showbiz reporter, and you can work with her on the story. She knows you'll be in touch.

I spent the night emailing Sarah as we worked on the article. The buzz reminded me of my time working in student journalism at university. It was exhilarating, exciting, and a familiar warm feeling settled in my stomach. Happy. I was happy.

I woke up the next morning to see the rest of the world had broken the story after *Metro*. A major tabloid had lifted my screenshots. However, Russell Crowe had responded to the accusation. I got back on Twitter, and messaged Gabe again with the update.

Thank you for all your spotting. Good work.

The original story got updated with the information I'd highlighted.

One good story wasn't enough; I needed another ...

The next day, I spotted an announcement from Eminem on social media.

Eminem's dropped a new track, by the way, I told Gabe on Twitter. His reply sent butterflies whooshing through my stomach.

Want to write the story?

Yeah, can do, I replied as nonchalantly as possible.

File a word / drive doc as quick as you can in Metro's tone and I'll run it through our system with your byline, he told me.

I listened to the track, and immediately knew what my headline was.

Eminem confirms new album and drops new track referring to Donald Trump as a 'loose cannon with his hand on the button'

The story went live an hour later.

A mutual friend of mine and Eli's messaged me out of the blue on Facebook a few days later.

Eli's been carrying a bag of your clothes around, crying on set at Channel 5.

I felt sick to my stomach. Most of my belongings I hadn't been able to carry had been clothes, mainly bras and underwear. Had he really been parading my knickers around at the TV show where we'd met?

They looked like crocodile tears. He turned them on the minute he saw me, wanting to know if I had any idea where you'd gone. He made me promise to ask you if you want the rest of your belongings.

I told her I didn't need anything, and that even if I could give out my address, I wouldn't run the risk of him finding it out.

When I told someone about it all later, they said something I reflected on for a long time.

'It's once they've lost that power over you and know they've lost that you start to see who they really are. Then you wonder how you were ever with them in the first place.'

A few weeks later, I was on the train home after an intense interview in Canary Wharf when I got a message on Twitter from Gabe.

Call me when you can.

Ten minutes later, I stood in a side street and dialled his number.

I didn't expect what was coming.

'I'd like to offer you the role of SEO reporter.'

'You haven't met me. Don't you want to say hi first?' I found myself saying.

'We can do that when we meet to discuss everything,' he replied. We arranged to meet the next day, and I hung up.

My mind was reeling. I was immediately cautious. I'd had a verbal offer to work in the media before, then had it taken away. I had to be prepared for that happening again.

The next day, I walked into Northcliffe House – where Metro.co.uk, Mail Online, the *Independent*, the I, and the *Evening Standard* are based – feeling so sick I was dizzy.

As I went in, I saw a man in a suit lying on a seat opposite me, shouting down the phone. And then Gabe appeared in front of me. It was strange. We'd been talking so much on Twitter, he felt more like a friend than my prospective employer. The conversation flowed, and to my surprise, I managed to keep my cool. 'Essentially, you're what we're looking for. A young journalist who knows what she's doing,' he told me.

After the meeting, I wandered through High Street Kensington towards the Tube, my head spinning. I'd done it. The pain was over. My life in London was about to begin.

CHAPTER 18

I'M REALLY HERE

I was out of training and ready to start my first day at Metro. Everything in my new workplace was so shiny and grand. I could hardly believe that I was in a professional newsroom, earning money. After a month or two, I'd be able to move out, get an ordinary rental. Life was going to get back to normal.

Shaking slightly with nerves, I took a seat. I looked at the computer in front of me and suddenly felt immobilised with fear. How was I going to do this? It felt like I was having an out of body experience. Was I really here? It felt like just yesterday I was lying on a filthy mattress. Now I was in my dream job. Could I actually do the work? What if I was rubbish and got fired? I tried not to hyperventilate and counted to 10.

'Um, I'm used to Macs, what do I need to do?' I managed to blurt out.

'Okay, I'll log you on,' Gabe said, grabbing the keyboard and starting to type. As I watched him load up my monitor, I gave myself an internal pep talk. Get it together! Don't screw this up before you've even started. He likes you. He thinks you're talented. Prove it. I took a drink and sat up straight. Right. I could do this.

*

'That was a good first week,' Gabe said on Friday afternoon, as I packed up my bag and got to my feet. I smiled.

'Thank you, it's been fun.'

'Now, next week, I won't be here, but Deb will show you the ropes. That is, if you're coming back.' He winked.

'I mean, I will on one condition. You follow me on Twitter,' I blurted out without thinking. It had been an ongoing joke – he was very picky about who he had on his social media.

My colleagues laughed. 'Looks like you're screwed, Gabe,' Deb added, and he laughed too. I smiled again. I felt warm inside. I belonged somewhere. People wanted to be around me. It felt strange, and I was exhausted, but I didn't feel so alone anymore.

*

As the months rolled on, I settled into London life for the first time. I got the Tube to work each day and felt like I was part of the commuter crowd, not some nobody on the fringe, pretending to be one of them. I got talking to other people in the newsroom, and wrote lifestyle articles, entertainment articles. It didn't feel like a job, because I was doing what I loved every day.

My boss, Deb, understood when things were hard for me and my PTSD flared up. I'd been writing a diary documenting my move to London, and I shared it with her. She read it, and it meant the world to know someone had heard my story. She encouraged me to write on varied topics, let me come up with new ideas, and supported me when I was feeling down. To this day, she remains a good friend.

When I got back to the refuge each evening after work, I didn't feel so empty anymore. I knew I had the safe haven of work to go to five times a week. Somewhere I belonged. And I was earning money, so I could start buying things for myself again.

The weekends brought with them a sense of peace and relaxation. Instead of melting into the vast chasm of time, I made the most of living in a quiet Zone 5 London suburb and went for long walks, taking in my surroundings and appreciating just how good it felt to be present in the moment. And I liked that. Being me felt good. It was a rare feeling, and I seized it with an overwhelming feeling of joy that I had never experienced before.

*

2017 dawned, and brought with it the experience of a lifetime. Monica, the travel editor, would email press trips around on a regular basis, and one of them in particular caught my eye. It was a trip to Reykjavik, Iceland, to cover a music festival. I hit reply immediately, and got booked on.

When my supervisor confirmed I could take the time off, I let excitement surge through me. It felt scary to be excited, and to have something to look forwards to, because I was so used to something going wrong. But a part of me said it was okay to feel that way, and so I let myself Google the places we'd be visiting and count down the days until my flight.

*

When we landed in Iceland, it felt like we were in another world. Our car took us down a desolate motorway with huge, ancient mountains quietly looming in the background. As I took in the unspoiled, ancient landscape, I felt truly privileged to be there. It was one of the most beautiful places in the world.

My hotel room had an incredible view of Reykjavik itself, but I wanted to soak up the atmosphere properly. So I plugged in my headphones and wandered down the steep, winding road.

It was starting to get dark, and the pastel-coloured houses were bathed in a warm glow. In the background, snow-capped mountains sat silently, as they had done for thousands of years. I kept walking until I reached Harpa, the distinctive concert hall that was emitting a quietly enchanting light show, the coloured glass reflecting onto the water.

I sat down on the wall overlooking the harbour, and breathed in the sea air. The rock-covered beach was adorned with stone towers, and beyond the vast expanse of water I could see the clouds drifting over the ancient mountains. It was breathtaking.

As I watched the waves ripple over the rocks and took in the beauty of what lay before me, I realised that I could never have imagined my life turning out this way. Just a few months ago, I'd been unemployed, homeless, and getting abused. Now I was a national journalist out in Reykjavik to cover a music festival. Although it would take a long time for all of my sadness to leave me, as I sat overlooking the harbour that night, I felt a piece of it fade away.

*

We spent four days out in Reykjavik, exploring the city and its surrounding areas by day and raving to experimental electronica in Harpa by night. I was exhausted upon my return to London, but it was the best kind of tiredness possible. I thought that would be the last of my trips for a while. It had certainly been the best break I'd ever had, but before too long, the perks of my career provided me with another once-in-a-lifetime experience ...

We're looking for people to come on a girls-only trip to Vegas, the PR email read, and I was allowed the five days off. The email detailing my flight across the Atlantic made my jaw drop. It cost *how much*?! And I was getting this whole trip free?!

Then the itinerary came through.

The Chainsmokers live at a poolside club.

Helicopter flight over Vegas.

Backstreet Boys live.

Magic Mike live.

Makeover and photoshoot at Seven Magic Mountains.

I couldn't imagine that all this stuff was being given to me. Why did I deserve it?

Life had been so filled with trauma and despair until that point in my life that I struggled to believe I'd be allowed these experiences. I was waiting for someone to send me an email, or step out from behind a secret door, and go 'Ha ha, just kidding you've been Punk'd.' Knowing my luck, they wouldn't even let me in the country ...

It took ages to get through immigration, and once I grabbed my bag, security stopped me on my way out.

'You've got everything you need in that bag?' the guard asked me.

'Um, yes,' I said, feeling scared. Oh, God. This was the bad luck I'd been waiting for. It was happening.

'Alright, I'm gonna need to check your bag, ma'am,' he said, taking me to one side. The other three girls were at the exit. I felt a sense of dread seep over me. I was never going to see America. I was going to get put straight on a plane back home. This was it.

'Where are your heels? You can't fit more than a pair or two in there,' he told me.

'Er, I travel light,' I told him.

'Alright, you're good. Welcome to Vegas,' he said, winking at me. Relief swept through me, and I ran out to join the others.

The heat hit me like a blanket the minute the airport's air conditioning disappeared. It dropped onto my entire body, smothering me and making it hard to breathe. I checked the weather app on my phone. It was 40 degrees Celsius. Oh ... my ... God.

We checked in at the hotel, and the attendant took a double take when he saw our names. 'Oh my gosh, press? You want water? Yeah? We have water,' he said, grabbing a load of bottles and throwing them at us. I laughed.

An hour later, I'd finished running around my massive room squealing with excitement at how amazing the view was, and how big my bed was. The huge bath and shower set-up was bigger than some of the rooms I'd slept in. And I screamed in disbelief upon opening my welcome pack and seeing a $200 gift card.

It was time to drink rum and watch some strippers.

We met up with the American and Canadian journalists on the way, and were ushered into the joint, where we got offered cocktails the size of our heads. Suddenly, we jumped as pounding music started blaring through the room. The show had begun.

By the end of it, we were being treated to lap dances and feeling both jet-lagged and drunk. We stumbled out to the minibus, and our guide screeched, 'Welcome to Vegas!'

We all screamed back in response as we got driven through the city. It was six o'clock in the morning UK time, but I was surrounded by the buzz of Vegas nightlife. I'd never felt so alive. *I made it,* I thought. *I'm really here.*

CHAPTER 19

CALIFORNIA

The months flew by, and before long, I realised I'd been living in London for two years. I'd switched jobs and become an editor, so my days were hectic and tiring. I lived with some annoying flatmates ... but I could lock my bedroom door, stretch out in bed, and relax in my own little happy place.

I was lonely, though.

Since uni had ended, I hadn't had many friends, and moving across the country, then going into an industry where I often worked erratic, unsociable hours, meant there wasn't much chance to make any new ones. Sometimes I used hook-up apps to meet guys, just because a one-night stand was better than spending every single night alone. I wasn't desperate for a romantic relationship, as I'd become quite used to enjoying my own company – but I did want to spend time with people at least occasionally, and sex was much quicker to obtain than genuine friendship. So, I downloaded Tinder, Bumble, and various other apps, and kept the bulk of my human contact outside work to digital messages or fleeting nights with strangers.

*

'Hi, I love your hair!'

I smiled as I saw the message. I got a fair amount of messages on Tinder. That wasn't a good thing, though – mostly it was men being explicit.

Checking my profile, I realised I hadn't included a bio, so this David guy had just gone with whatever he could work with. I checked his profile. Beard. Works with robots. Cute bunny. 'Have a high-power blender, so date me if you love hummus and Oreo milkshakes.'

I was sold. I messaged him back, and the conversation flowed. Screenshotting an extract and sending it to a friend, she was surprised. 'You're never that enthusiastic with anyone! This guy must be really special.'

'I guess so ...' I had no idea how it had happened. I was a fast texter, and so was he. Within a few days, barely an hour went by where we weren't messaging each other. Talking to him felt as natural as breathing. But the more we bonded, first over the little things – what we were up to, how bored we were at work – then moving into the deeper stuff, the more we both got scared. This conversation was so perfect, it felt like glass. It could shatter at any moment. Especially when we addressed the elephant in the room – meeting up in real life.

Although we openly admitted our fears to each other, I felt like something else had to be said. 'I'm not exactly a Size Zero model,' I hesitantly typed, looking down at my flabby stomach and sighing. My self-esteem wasn't exactly sky-high. But after a few weeks of talking to David, it felt like we were best friends, and if he had suddenly disappeared from my life, it would have seriously hurt. It felt strange, and slightly worrying, to be so affected by a person I'd known for less than a month and hadn't even met in person. But I was already in too deep.

My work schedule was hectic, but we eventually found an evening when we were both free. He booked a table at a restaurant in Shoreditch, and when he sent a link to the menu online, I started getting butterflies in my stomach.

I'd never been on a real date before. When I'd been with Jasper, we had spent all of our time in his room, occasionally venturing outside for a brief walk. Due to lack of funds, our rare trips out were usually with Kate, who paid for everything, so we could never really talk or do anything romantic. Now, though, I was going to dinner with someone I really liked. And I was scared shitless.

'Let's have a phone call before we meet,' I suddenly said one night. He agreed, and I called him without thinking about it. His voice was warm, intelligent, and inquisitive, and we stayed on the phone for two hours. Several times, I was laughing so hard my stomach hurt. When I hung up, I had a huge smile on my face.

After work the following night, I got changed in the toilets, feeling jittery. *I have to just do it, and if he doesn't like me, it's not going to kill me,* I thought, forcing myself back out of the cubicle and out into the night.

Sitting at Liverpool Street station, I pretended I was deeply absorbed in my phone so I didn't have to look around and potentially miss seeing him coming. I wanted to look cool, independent, and relaxed, not a bag of nerves desperately awaiting his arrival. *Calm the hell down*, I told myself. I didn't.

Suddenly, he was in front of me. Straightaway the conversation flowed just as it had online. Dinner was delicious, and as I watched him talk, occasionally smiling, I saw his lips curling upwards into a goofy grin, and felt a twinge in my stomach.

When we kissed, it felt as if we'd been doing it for years, and when I said goodbye, we immediately started messaging again, planning the next time we could meet.

The two weeks that followed were blissful. Until that point, my life had consisted of working round-the-clock shifts, followed by a collapse into exhausted sleep. But instead, I would head over to David's flat. He always got me the food I liked, and I'd look forwards to chilling in front of the TV, with his arm around me, and his animals running around at my feet. It wasn't long before I was staying overnight, his quiet, luxurious place was so much nicer than my dodgy rental in East London.

But one night at four o'clock in the morning, everything changed.

A buzzer jolted me awake, sending a cold fear through my stomach. David got to his feet and headed to the front door to see who it was. He came back to me, looking rattled.

'This is going to sound really weird, but my psycho ex is here, and I need to go and deal with her.' He put his shoes on and closed the door. Another shot of fear seared through me as I heard the key turn in the lock.

Why was he locking me in?

I jumped out of bed, suddenly wide awake, and headed to the balcony. Could I leave that way if there was a fire? No, it was locked. Shit!

David's cat woke up and ran to my feet, mewing. I sat on the sofa with him, mindlessly stroking him and feeling jumpy. Why had he locked me in? Did he think this "psycho ex" was dangerous? Did he suddenly not want me to leave? Was this all some plot to trap me there? I started hyperventilating and had to try to force myself to calm down, before I contacted him. I messaged to ask if everything was okay. No reply. Time stood still for a while.

Staring at a spot on the wall, I wondered what was going on. What if he didn't come back? How would I leave? I had to work the night shift later. What if I was trapped?

An hour later, he replied, telling me she was refusing to leave and threatening to call the police. Once he finally came back upstairs, he apologised for dragging me into the drama. 'I can drive you home if you want,' he offered.

'Well, if you think she's going to come back here and give you grief, why don't we just go and sleep at my place?'

He put his head on my chest and I wrapped my arms around him. He thanked me for being so accommodating, and said he'd bring the car around.

'Please don't lock me in here again, that was a dick move. What if there had been a fire?'

He handed me his flat key and left, going around the back so he didn't run into her on the way out.

A few minutes later, the door rattled. I assumed it was David, trying to get back in. But then my phone pinged with a message from him. It simply said: *She tricked me. She's here.* My heart dropped to my stomach. It wasn't David at the door; she was trying to get in? Who was this crazy bitch?

The door rattled again, and I ran into the bedroom, slamming the door shut. What the fuck would I do if she came in here? I dialled 999 and locked my phone screen in case I had to suddenly call the cops. Maybe I should call them anyway ...

The door opened, and my heart started thumping in my chest. I froze when a voice called out my name, then relaxed when I recognised David's voice. I opened the bedroom door.

'She was waiting outside so that when I left, she could get in. I think she's going to come in when I open the door again. Will you run with me?'

Will you run with me? What the hell was happening? Why was I suddenly running away from some crazy woman with the guy I'd met on Tinder just a few weeks ago? But what choice did I have? If I didn't, she would just come in and God knew what would happen next.

I just nodded mutely, pulled on my shoes, grabbed my bag, and took his hand. The door opened, and a woman barrelled into the room, heading straight for the bedroom. David dragged me out, slamming the door shut behind him, and we hurried outside.

Now that I was safely out in the open, the crisp night air returned me to my senses. The fear quickly subsided, and my mind went into overdrive. I started firing off questions.

'What is she going to do in there?'

'Probably just sleep. At worst, she'll break some stuff.'

'She's done this before?' He nodded, brow furrowed. There was something he wasn't telling me. I frowned.

'So, if she's done this before, why haven't you called the police? She's breaking and entering right now. It's against the law. And if she breaks stuff, that's criminal damage! Why are we running away from her? Don't let her drive you out of your own home, call the cops!'

David was shaking his head, looking exhausted. There was a weariness in his eyes that told me the history behind the story he wasn't telling me ran long and deep; that it was locked away in his mind and he'd only reveal tiny details as it became absolutely necessary.

'The police always take the woman's side. It's easier to just let her stay there.'

Something wasn't adding up. I started walking back inside.

'Where are you going?'

'I need to find out what she's doing in there. I need to call the police. If I call them, and tell them she just turned up, they can kick her out.'

'Can't we just leave?' David looked tortured, pleading. I was beginning to get very suspicious. What the hell was he hiding from me? I felt a strange pull towards the flat. I had to go back inside, because the answers to this mystery would unravel once I spoke to this woman.

I marched through the door, with David trailing behind me, and saw the woman sitting on the bed. She looked perfectly at home.

'David, what the fuck? Who is this?'

Then she said something that made my blood run cold.

'We're married, you can't just give me notice to vacate.' I noticed an American twang to her accent.

I froze. 'You're married.' It was a statement, not a question. I wasn't sure who to believe. But this woman was calm and collected, and David was panicking. It looked like his web of lies was crumbling around him.

'I kicked you out on Friday! I told you to leave, multiple times!'

'But we're married, I legally live here.'

David turned to me. 'It was just for a visa, I told her to leave and she refuses.'

The woman got up. 'I don't know who this is, and if you want to cheat on me, do it. Have a girlfriend, whatever, but you can't lock me out.'

She turned to look at me. 'What are you doing here?'

'I'm just … trying to understand the situation.'

'I think you should leave.'

'Yeah … I think I should.' I turned around and walked to the lift. David ran after me. 'Imi, wait!'

I looked up at him; watched him search for words to say, then give up. He got into the lift with me.

'Get out.'

The words came out in a controlled growl. I was shocked at the amount of anger in my voice. I couldn't feel anything right now. But on some other, subconscious level, I was clearly seething.

David looked at me and knew I meant business. He got out and looked at me. 'Will I ever talk to you again?'

'No.' The lift doors closed, and I was gone.

*

I closed my bedroom door behind me. The sun was just starting to rise. I felt empty. For the last few weeks, the room had just been the place I threw my stuff into before rushing off to David's place. Now that was over, this was all I had left.

Running on autopilot, I got undressed and into bed. It was six o'clock in the morning. I had a shift at two o'clock. I briefly considered calling in sick, then decided I wasn't going to do that. I had a life to maintain. Much as I hated the situation, I couldn't just opt out. Opting out would have left me with nothing; I needed to keep going through the motions, get money in my bank account, keep a roof over my head.

One day things would change, and I'd thought they might change with David, but I'd been a fool. He was married. He was … married. He had a wife. It was all lies. Everything he'd told me was a lie.

I curled up into a ball and cried myself to sleep.

*

'What a dick.'

'Just forget about him, he's not worth it.'

'Seriously? You deserve so much better.'

'Forget he existed.'

My phone vibrated again. It wasn't an online friend this time. It was David.

'I wasn't trying to lie to you, it wasn't really a marriage.'

'She refuses to take her stuff and is trying to insist she still lives here because of it.'

'But all that said, I do understand if you never want to talk to me again.'

'She's just trying to make it seem like we were together because she's still trying to be with me despite me breaking up with her and reaffirming it on many occasions. But rather than deal with it, she's trying to get rid of you.'

'Just know that regardless of what happens now, I meant what I said about you. And I hope that even if it can't be with me anymore that you can be comfortable with someone. Sorry.'

All the words swirled around my head. I didn't know what to think anymore. I watched my online friends message me advice, and didn't know how to reply. I did my job, I ate, I slept. I trusted my mind to work on it. At some point, it would produce an answer.

*

'I still want to be friends with you.'

David looked up at me in shock. We were sitting in a shopping centre near Canary Wharf. I nursed my coffee mug.

'I can't just cut you out of my life. I've been drifting through life for years now, not really sure where I'm going or who I am. I just do this journalism thing because it's what pays the bills, but I don't know what really makes me happy. You made me happy. And you lied to me, and you destroyed my trust, and I know that whatever you tell me about Jess could be a lie to save your ass, but I'll hear you out, and I'll weigh it up, and we'll spend time together. But obviously all the physical stuff is over. It's just over.'

He smiled. 'Thank you for giving me a second chance. It's more than I deserve.'

I wondered if I was doing the right thing. I'd put trust in people before, and it had gone horribly wrong. What if the same thing happened again?

But then I realised I'd rather take the risk than spend the rest of my life wondering what could have been.

*

'We're here.'

David pulled up outside the hotel. Everything was so quiet. I looked around in wonder.

'It's so beautiful here.'

'Well, I want this to be special. It's your birthday, after all.'

It was mid-April, a sunny Saturday afternoon, and we'd just driven for five hours up to the Lake District for my 25th birthday. The next three days stretched out ahead of me. No hectic shifts at work. No standing on a stuffy Underground line. It was just me, David, and so much green my head was spinning.

It had been a month since I'd let David back into my life. I'd told him he needed to tell me everything about his relationship with Jess, prove he was getting a divorce, and prove he was dedicated to me. He had obliged.

Four years ago, David had been browsing Reddit when he'd come across a post that had caught his eye. A woman, clearly drunk, was talking intelligently about all the things he loved to discuss. He messaged her, and before long they were close.

A few months later, he flew to Philadelphia to meet her, and they spent time together, realising they wanted to make a relationship work. It wasn't long before she flew to Jersey, the small island near France where David had grown up, and said she had nothing tying her to America. Much as he felt it was strange, he let her live with him, and because he wanted to get to know her more and not worry she'd have to go back overseas, he married her so she could stay in the UK.

'Are you fucking insane? That's not how you get to know someone,' I exclaimed, and he just said that sometimes in life, he took risks. 'If they work out, they work out, and if they don't, that's just life,' he said.

I frowned, and bit my tongue.

The first year or so was blissful, but by the time he'd moved to London to start a new job, her mental illness had begun to rear its head. A psychiatrist believed she had borderline personality disorder and elements of schizophrenia.

David told me, 'She refused to get a job. She just lay around, depressed, all the time. I tried to help her get therapy, see a doctor, but she didn't want to. She said she didn't trust them. I wanted to talk to her family, but she wouldn't let me.

'She cut me off from all my friends and family, she was paranoid I was seeing someone else; even had a go at me if I even talked to another woman. I started working long hours at the office, just to avoid her. Sometimes she would have funny turns, try to stab herself, stab me, run up and down the corridors screaming.

'She was obsessed with my exes. Would track them down. Threaten to burn down their homes. Threaten to burn down my office. She'd slip drugs into my drink.

'She's always on something. Xanax, speed, whatever she can get off the streets.

'For a while, her threats were earth-shattering to me. She'd say she wanted to go back to America, I'd pay for her plane ticket, she'd never go. She'd say she was going to leave me. For a while, I was devastated. But as time went on, I realised my feelings had grown less and less for her. Eventually, when she threatened to leave, I just told her that was fine. So she started threatening to kill herself instead.'

Left lonely and isolated, David had turned to Tinder, and met me. He hadn't told me all of this, because he'd been worried I'd run a mile. Jess had been staying in an Airbnb when I'd been seeing him, but she'd turned up out of the blue that night.

I wasn't sure what to believe. His story did add up, and if it was true, my heart went out to him, but ... 'What's the situation now?'

'The night she turned up, I slept on the sofa, then got a hotel for the rest of the week. When I went back to see if she was there, she was gone. She'd bagged up all her clothes and put them in bin bags by the door. She texts me every few weeks. As far as I know, she's in the Netherlands right now. Thinks she can start a new life over there.'

'On whose money?'

'I'm giving her £800 a month right now.'

I was incredulous. 'So your wife is wandering around the world on your money, texting and calling every month or so to beg to get back with you and threaten to kill herself?'

It was so much to take in. I thought for a while, then spoke again.

'This could take years. I just ... I would have to wait for you. You would have to prove yourself to me ...'

It was a commitment of sorts. I was making a commitment to him. I was willing to trust him. So, we tentatively resumed our relationship, with me feeling wary and paranoid whenever I wasn't with him. What if he was seeing her when I wasn't around? What if this was all a lie, and I was just his side chick?

But I couldn't worry about that. At the end of the day, I'd decided to pursue the relationship, despite my trust in him having nearly been destroyed. He made me happy, and my life was fuller with him. It was strange: for the first time in my life, I wasn't running away. I wasn't escaping from the situation when it had become too much for me, even when other people recommended that I ran and didn't look back.

Something inside me had become stronger. I wanted to see this through.

*

'It's so quiet here.'

We were lying in bed together, looking out at the night sky and talking.

'Have you had a good birthday?'

'The best. Thank you so much.' I rolled over and kissed him.

'Is it going to be shit to go back to your grotty room after this?' he asked.

I groaned slightly, thinking about walking into my room again, listening to trains rumble past and breathing in weed smoke. David held me tighter.

'You know, I didn't want to say this, because we've only known each other a few months, but I just wanted to say that, you know, I'm moving to my new place soon, and you can stay over as much as you want. And, if you were comfortable ... if you wanted to move in with me. Just for a few months, while you save up money for a place of your own. You can. And of course you can say no, or ignore everything I just said, or ...' He was rambling, much as he had the day he'd accidentally let slip an 'I love you' and turned bright red.

'I ... I need to think about it. It does make sense. But, you're right. I have only known you a few months. And even though Jess won't know where you are, what if she finds you? I can't go through her turning up at the door again.' But, a part of me thought, if I lived with him, I'd know for sure he wasn't secretly seeing her. Not a great foundation to start things off, though.

'Well, you can stay over as much as you want. It's only a 15-minute train journey to London Bridge, so it's convenient for your late shifts, too.'

I nodded, and was silent. I looked up at the painting on the wall opposite us. It was a big purple flower with dark green leaves on a dark backdrop. I liked it. It made me feel peaceful. But I was wary, too. I remembered all too well what had happened last time I moved in with someone I barely knew in London. What if David turned into someone else, like Eli had?

For the next few days, I weighed up the pros and cons in my head. A week later, I decided that once I'd saved up enough money for me to get out if things got bad, I'd move in with him. So I said yes. I ignored all the voices in my head telling me not to take the risk. But, as David himself had said to me, sometimes in life you've got to take risks. *If they work out, they work out, and if they don't, that's just life.*

I decided to plunge into life head first.

*

A month later

It was six o'clock in the evening, and the night sky was clear. David was still at work, and we were messaging online, discussing Jess. Again.

'I just don't know why she's still in the Netherlands. How much longer are you going to fund her to do whatever she likes?'

'I don't want her to refuse a divorce. I need to keep her in my good books.'

I sighed. 'How much could she screw you over in a settlement?'

There was silence for a few minutes. I figured he'd been called over by a colleague, or something. Then he typed a message.

'Fuck.'

'What?'

'I just got a call from a coroner in Mexico. And I swear this isn't a joke ...'

My mind immediately jumped to the correct conclusion. Oh, fuck. Fuck. Fuck.

'Jess killed herself in a hotel room in Tijuana. The coroner is asking me to claim the remains ...'

Was he ... joking? ... No, he wouldn't joke about something like that.

There was silence for a few minutes.

'I just got off the phone. I just need to focus on coming home. I'm coming home.'

I jumped to my feet. The bed needed making. It seemed like such a stupid thought under the circumstances, but I was obsessed with making the bed perfect, so he could lie on it when he came in. I added new bed sheets, plumped up the pillows, and straightened corners until I heard the key turn in the door.

The only time I'd seen David show much emotion was when Jess had turned up at his old flat, and he'd been arguing with her. He'd clearly become like that after years of being "taught" that showing emotion was somehow wrong.

From day to day, he didn't really show how he was feeling very much. Typical man, I sometimes thought. My sexy robot, I would joke to myself.

When he walked through the door that night, he was a mess. I'd never seen him like that. He was a broken man.

How much did he really love her, then? a snide voice hissed in my head. Then I kicked myself. His wife has just died! Put your own fucking feelings aside. He needs you.

He lay down on the bed and I held him while he cried. 'I'm pretty sure I know how she did it. I don't need to wait for the autopsy results. It was a drug overdose. She left my name and address in her suicide note. She killed herself on the day of our wedding anniversary. She'd always threatened to do it, for years, I just didn't think she'd actually do it ...

'What if she was in pain? What if she died a slow, painful death, blaming me? This is all my fault. I killed someone. I killed her ...'

I was out of my depth. I tried to compare the self-assured woman I'd seen a few months earlier, with the corpse lying on a hotel room bed in Mexico. It was impossible. And there was no way I could lie to him and tell him she hadn't gone blaming him. For all I knew, she had been so unable to move on from him that she'd decided the only way out was death. And she could have taken the wrong amount and been in agony until her final breath. I struggled for the right words to say, and held him until they came.

'You did so much for her. You helped someone for much longer than most people would have considered reasonable. You gave up most of your life for her. You offered her a lifeline not many people would be able to, because you had the funds to provide her therapy, rehab, whatever she needed.

'This was her choice. Her mental illness was clouding her, for her entire life, and she chose not to accept the help you gave her. Sometimes you can't fix everything. I know you wanted her to get better, but she made the choice not to. I know that doesn't make it better, but you need to remember this is not your fault. You did so much for her. She made the choice to go.'

He buried his head into my chest and sobbed. I held him and wondered what the hell was going to happen now.

A part of me felt like I knew what her life had been like. For nearly two decades, I'd spent my life running away when things became too tough. I'd put myself in dangerous situations, and sometimes I'd wondered if it was worth carrying on. But every time I considered opting out, I thought about what I'd be leaving behind. Not just family and friends, but hopes and dreams. And when things had been hard, I had held on to the belief that they would get better. *This too shall pass*, read the tattoo on my left arm.

And I had moved past it. I'd found other ways to cope with the confusing mess in my head. Sometimes it was hard, sometimes I said and did things I regretted, and I'd lost so many friends due to my erratic behaviour. It hurt, but I kept looking forwards. There was always a way forwards.

David told me that Jess had dreamt of going into medicine. I thought about the Jess who could have been a top doctor, saving lives, then compared her to the one who had taken her own. I realised it could so easily have been me. I could have been the one lying in a hotel room, in a ditch, in the river. But I wasn't. I was still here.

I felt grateful for the life I'd given myself, and cried for the life Jess would never have.

Two weeks later

Just a few months earlier, I'd been in a boring routine of riding the Underground, sitting in an office and going to Tesco to pick up ready meals for one. Now I was on a crazy ride across the world, about to ride in a Mustang down to San Diego and then hop over the border to Mexico, so we could get David's estranged wife cremated.

After a tense few days of waiting for the Mexican coroner to call every evening, contacting the US Embassy to get them to go down to the morgue and identify Jess's body, and seeing the chilling photos they'd emailed over of her tattoos so he could confirm it was her, he'd made the decision to fly out to the US and take care of it.

I wanted to be there, too, in case he needed me. I didn't want him to have to go through it alone.

*

'Oh wow, I thought those palm trees were only in movies.'

Dave was revving up the Mustang, while I stretched out in the passenger seat, sunglasses on. David looked over at me.

'When this is over, life will go back to normal, I promise. I just want to be with you and enjoy our life together. I don't think I'll ever be the same after what's happened, but maybe we can both be a bit broken together. I just want to be happy, and I think you do too.'

I kissed him. 'Let's do this.'

He pulled out into the road, and we sped through the blazing sunshine towards the highway.

CHAPTER 20

REFLECTIONS OF A MAD TRAVELLER

Once David and I got back from California, life settled into a routine. It got easier, with time. It's not all fixed yet. What would that look like, anyway? But things are okay.

David makes me happy, and I have hope that as he heals from the most traumatic event of his life, I will get to see more of the person he once was.

As for me ... I'm alright, you know? Sometimes life gets hard, but that's how it is for everyone. I didn't go through what I did, expecting that it would be a bed of roses on the other side. I just wanted something normal. And I've got that.

Things are up and down. I have bad patches. I'm not going to pretend I'm fully functioning, 100 percent of the time. I'm not. Sometimes, I'm a mess. As I write this, I've managed to mess things up with a job I loved, and I'm feeling a bit lost again. But I talk to the people close to me, I save my money, I think of ways I can move forwards, and I know that I can get through it.

I sometimes find it hard to believe that my life really panned out the way it did. I read back over this book, and huge chunks of it don't feel real. But I know it is.

Many people will probably want to know why I held on so stubbornly to the hell I went through in London, when I could have just gone home. Well, there's no easy answer to this one. I knew that if I went home, I would have been incredibly unlikely to get back into the capital – the only place I felt I could get a decent career in my industry. My parents wanted me to work entry-level jobs and work my way into journalism. But I know that's not always how these things work. There just weren't enough entry-level jobs, and those that were around wouldn't hire me, suspecting I wouldn't stay there for long.

Working my way into journalism would have required somehow funding a postgraduate degree. Many of my peers from university had rich parents who could do that. I didn't meet the requirements for a loan, and I'm not convinced my dad would have been able to give me the money.

I know I made mistakes. I know I acted recklessly. But it's easy to look back over the past and pick out things you would have done better, once you have the wisdom to know differently. I was young, clouded with mental illness, and just wanted to be happy. I went through hell, made a lot of rash decisions, but I wouldn't change a thing. I'm proud of who I am today. Yes, I'm overweight, and yes, I have a nicotine addiction. But really? It could have been a lot worse.

My Mad Traveller is largely dormant now. I constantly have a niggling background fear that she will come back. I have seizures, sometimes. I see and hear things, from time to time. Sometimes, I will wake up in the middle of the night, feeling like I can't cope. I will hyperventilate, start sweating, and start planning to run away. The Mad Traveller floats out of her Cupboard, ghost-like, and I think about how I could book a plane ticket to New Zealand, go and live in the mountains, not deal with getting up early every morning to go to work, busy Underground trains, obnoxious members of the public, paying the bills, maintaining a relationship ...

One Sunday afternoon a few months ago, I told David how I felt sometimes. 'I think we all want to run away, sometimes,' he told me, and I was surprised.

'If shit ever hits the fan, I'll get on that plane to New Zealand with you. Fuck it.'

I suddenly remembered one of the many times I'd briefly run away from school. I was about 14 and chose to hide in the bushes down the road for several hours. My dad had found me, and I felt ashamed because he'd had to take time off work to come and find me. He sat down next to me in the bushes and told me he felt like I did, sometimes.

'Do you think I want to get up and go to work every day, go to endless meetings, deal with clients and pay bills? I don't. I'd much rather be home with you. My family. But I know I have responsibilities. I want you all to be well fed, clothed, kept warm, and to have futures. So, I go out, and I work, because I know that's what I have to do. I know it's hard, Imi, but whenever you feel like you can't cope, all you have to do is talk to me.'

Sometimes, when I wake up in the middle of the night, I cuddle into David as he sleeps, or go out to the lounge, where my kitten will run up to me, nuzzling into me and mewing. I have my own little family now, and I wouldn't give it up for the world.

In some ways, everyone has their own Mad Traveller, lying within them, threatening to come out and play whenever life becomes too much. Sometimes we go and take a drive after an argument, imagining we could just keep going, set up a new life in another town, and start again. Sometimes we have a panic attack and struggle to breathe. Sometimes we lie curled up in bed alone, sobbing. But it's not those feelings that define us. It's what we choose to do with those feelings, and the life we create, that makes us who we really are. And after several years of being defined by my Mad Traveller, I feel that now, my life is my own.

To everyone who struggles to get through the day-to-day – you're not alone. Life is hard. It's a rollercoaster. But staying on the ride is always worth it.

CHAPTER 21

AFTERWORD

'Alright, are you ready?' Lucy asked, standing at the door.

'Yup, good to go,' I replied. Luke nodded.

There were 60 or 70 students in the lecture theatre. The room felt so familiar, yet so different. I remembered entering it for the first time, a timid 19-year-old university student, and sitting hesitantly on the back row, feeling scared and unsure of myself.

Now I was on the other side – standing before rows of expectant faces, who had signed up to hear me give a speech about how to get into journalism.

Luke and I had tossed a coin before heading down, and determined that he'd go first. So I sat back for the first 20 minutes and watched him talk to the crowd. They laughed at the right times, scribbled down notes, and eagerly raised their hands to ask questions at the end.

Then Luke was sitting down, I was getting to my feet, and all eyes were on me ...

A jolt of fear shot through me. Could I do this? Would I stumble over my words, make a fool of myself? What did I know about getting into journalism? They deserved better than me. I should just walk out, now ... Or so went the dialogue in my head – but I wasn't listening.

I took a seat in front of the crowd, put my laptop down in front of me, and glanced down at my speech.

'I'll probably just be staring at this screen, reading off it, just so you know,' I said. I paused. I had expected my voice to sound shaky, but it didn't. My voice sounded clear, confident. Powerful, even. I looked up, and looked again at the faces who gazed back at me. They weren't so scary.

I put the laptop away. I didn't need notes. I knew exactly what to say.

I smiled, took a deep breath, and began to speak.

*

There was a time when I was a quiet little girl who didn't know how to talk to anyone. I sat in the corner, on my own, reading a book. I avoided social contact, and got scared incredibly easily. I didn't like being alone, but it was better than having to face real life.

Now that I'm older, I've realised life isn't meant to be easy. Sometimes I have to take a deep breath before I walk out of my front door, but I'm not scared anymore.

I've had good experiences and bad over the years. Things are still a little uncertain for me, but I prefer it that way. I don't want to be bored, and I want to be continually challenging myself, becoming more aware of myself and what makes me happy.

I'm grateful to my previous managers – two powerful women, who showed me such compassion when I needed it most. They taught me how to harness my best qualities and inspire others. To my surprise, I've managed to keep doing the latter, even when I don't believe I'm the best version of myself.

Speaking freestyle to a room full of strangers is proof that I'm no longer the shy little girl who ran away from everything. The audience laughed at my jokes, and laughed some more when I hadn't even realised I was being funny. It made me feel good about myself.

I've still got a long way to go, but the difference now is that I believe I will achieve what I want to, in the end. I'm not running away anymore, I'm running towards whatever the future brings me.

ACKNOWLEDGEMENTS

I'd like to thank Cameron, for offering his support unconditionally from the start. Who'd have thought I'd be running across a road in Mexico to reach a Walmart toilet just three months after meeting you ... or breezing down the highway in California on three hours' sleep. Or cuddling into a brand-new kitten, my heart filled with love. You taught me that I can be happy again, and I don't have to be scared of talking about my mental health. Thank you.

To Deb, also, for listening to the beginnings of my story back in the *Metro* days. Without your support – and you saving my ass, repeatedly, emotionally, and financially, every time I screwed up – I wouldn't be as strong as I am now. Thank you. Your insight and wisdom is invaluable.

To Chris at Trigger, for helping me shape my story into the best version possible – and helping me to draw out parts that I'd left buried in my mind for a long time. You have helped me realise the dream I held as a little girl – to one day be holding a book with my name on it.

To Dan, Elliott, and Jonn – we only talk online, now, but I know you've got my back whenever I need it. We've seen a fair amount of shit together, and I'm glad you were there through it all. Thank you for putting up with my crazy.

Last, but not least. Dad, I love you. It took a while for us to really start talking, but we got there in the end.

**If you found this book interesting ...
why not read these next?**

Unbroken

Learning to Live Beyond My Diagnosis

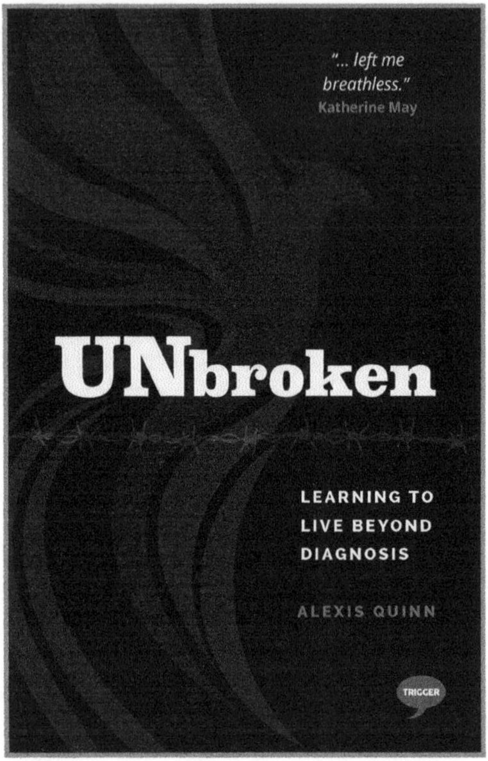

Unbroken tells the story of a woman misdiagnosed after succumbing to grief when her brother died. After years of fighting a label that did not fit, she finally found escape.

Sex, Suicide and Serotonin

Taking Myself Apart, Putting Myself Back Together

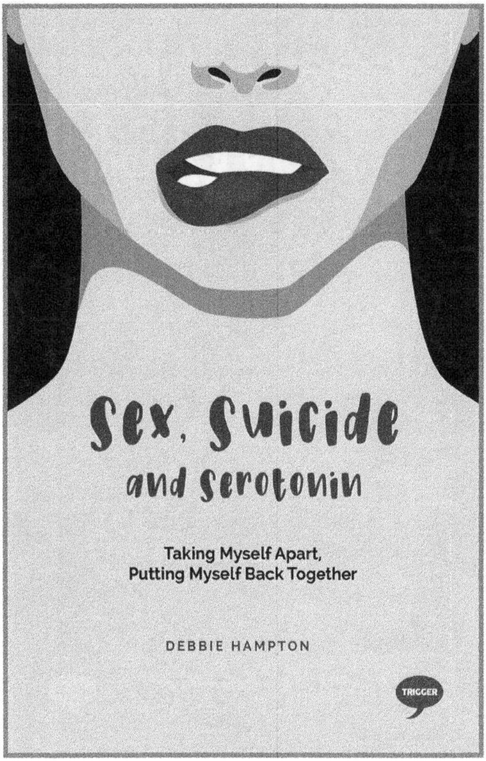

When Debbie took a near-lethal mix of wine and drugs, she didn't want to wake up – but she did. Here Debbie tells the story of how she forged a new life.

Walk a Mile

Tales of a Wandering Loon

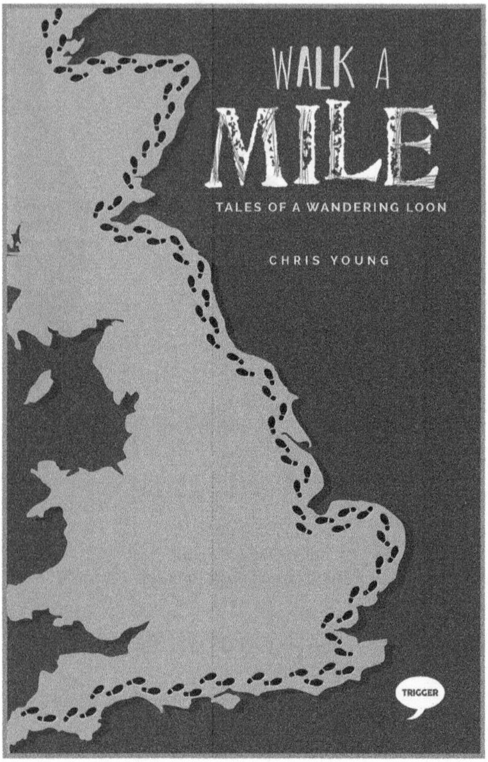

This is the story of Chris Young, a sufferer of BPD, who decided to walk around the edge of the UK, challenging mental health stigma one conversation at a time.

the Shaw mind
FOUNDATION

Creating hope for children, adults and families

Sign up to our charity, The Shaw Mind Foundation

www.shawmindfoundation.org

and keep in touch with us; we would love to hear from you.

We aim to bring to an end the suffering and despair caused by mental health issues. Our goal is to make help and support available for every single person in society, from all walks of life. We will never stop offering hope. These are our promises.

TRIGGER™

The voice of mental health

www.triggerpublishing.com

Trigger is a publishing house devoted to opening conversations about mental health. We tell the stories of people who have suffered from mental illnesses and recovered, so that others may learn from them.

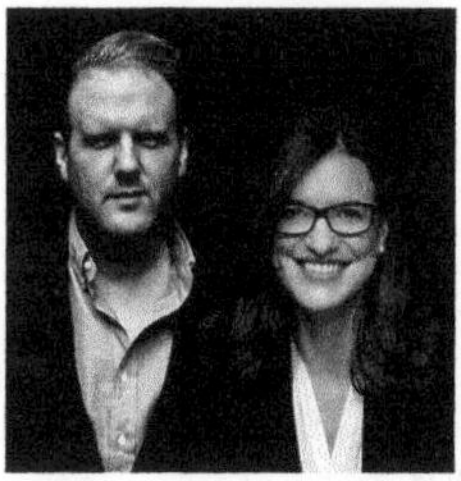

Adam Shaw is a worldwide mental health advocate and philanthropist. Now in recovery from mental health issues, he is committed to helping others suffering from debilitating mental health issues through the global charity he co-founded, The Shaw Mind Foundation. www.shawmindfoundation.org

Lauren Callaghan (CPsychol, PGDipClinPsych, PgCert, MA (hons), LLB (hons), BA), born and educated in New Zealand, is an innovative industry-leading psychologist based in London, United Kingdom. Lauren has worked with children and young people, and their families, in a number of clinical settings providing evidence based treatments for a range of illnesses, including anxiety and obsessional problems. She was a psychologist at the specialist national treatment centres for severe obsessional problems in the UK and is renowned as an expert in the field of mental health, recognised for diagnosing and successfully treating OCD and anxiety related illnesses in particular. In addition to appearing as a treating clinician in the critically acclaimed and BAFTA award-winning documentary *Bedlam*, Lauren is a frequent guest speaker on mental health conditions in the media and at academic conferences. Lauren also acts as a guest lecturer and honorary researcher at the Institute of Psychiatry Kings College, UCL.